WALL PILATES

WORKOUTS FOR WOMEN

Transform Your Body and Your Life with Julia - Step-by-Step Videos and Photo Illustrations, Easy to Follow & Low-Impact. A 28-Day Challenge Guide for All - Beginner to Advanced Workout Plans Included.

JULIA SUNNYFLOW

Acknowledgment

I would like to express my sincere gratitude to all those who have contributed to the creation of this book.

Special thanks to my family and friends for their unwavering support, encouragement, and understanding throughout this journey.

I also want to express my appreciation to the Pilates community for their inspiration, passion, and commitment to wellness.

Lastly, to you, dear reader, thank you for embarking on this journey with me. May this book empower and inspire you to embrace the transformative power of Wall Pilates in your life.

With gratitude,

Julia Sunnyflow

© Copyright 2024 – by Julia Sunnyflow – All Rights Reserved.

Table of Contents

INTRODUCTION

Welcome to the beginning of a transformative journey, where the walls around you are not barriers, but pathways to strength, flexibility, and profound well-being. In the pages ahead, we'll delve into the realm of Wall Pilates—a dynamic fusion of traditional Pilates principles and innovative wall-based exercises designed specifically for women seeking a holistic approach to fitness.

Origins and History

The origins and history of Wall Pilates are intertwined with the evolution of Joseph Pilates' original method—a revolutionary approach to fitness and rehabilitation that continues to inspire and empower individuals worldwide. To comprehend the origins of Wall Pilates, it is crucial to delve into the intricate history of Pilates and examine how this inventive approach evolved as a seamless continuation of its fundamental principles.

Joseph Pilates, a German-born visionary, developed his method in the early 20th century with a profound understanding of the interconnectedness between mind, body, and spirit. Drawing inspiration from disciplines as diverse as gymnastics, yoga, and martial arts, Pilates sought to create a holistic system of exercise that would promote strength, flexibility, and overall well-being.

The early years of Pilates' career were marked by innovation and experimentation as he honed his method and refined his approach to movement and rehabilitation. During World War I, Pilates was interned in a prisoner-of-war camp, where he began to develop his exercises using improvised equipment to help fellow detainees maintain their physical and mental health. It was here that the seeds of his method were sown, laying the groundwork for what would later become known as Pilates.

Upon his release from the camp, Pilates immigrated to the US, where he founded the first Pilates studio in New York City in the 1920s. Initially embraced by dancers and athletes for its ability to improve performance and prevent injury, Pilates' method gradually gained recognition as a transformative approach to fitness for people of all ages and abilities.

Over the decades that followed, Pilates' method continued to evolve as his students and followers adapted and expanded upon his original teachings. The principles of control, concentration, precision, and breath became the guiding tenets of the Pilates philosophy, shaping the way practitioners approached each exercise and movement.

It was against this backdrop of innovation and evolution that Wall Pilates began to take shape. As Pilates enthusiasts sought new ways to deepen their practice and challenge their bodies, the idea of incorporating a wall into Pilates exercises emerged as a natural progression. The wall provided a stable surface for support and resistance, allowing practitioners to explore movements with greater control and precision.

The concept of Wall Pilates gained momentum in the late 20th century, thanks in part to the pioneering efforts of fitness instructors and movement therapists who recognized its potential to enhance the traditional Pilates repertoire. By incorporating the wall into familiar exercises such as the Hundred, the Roll-Up, and the Swan, practitioners discovered new dimensions of strength, stability, and alignment.

In recent years, Wall Pilates has experienced a resurgence in popularity as more women seek alternative approaches to fitness that prioritize functionality, sustainability, and holistic well-being. With its emphasis on core strength, postural alignment, and mindful movement, Wall Pilates offers a refreshing departure from traditional gym-based workouts, inviting women to connect more deeply with their bodies and cultivate a greater sense of self-awareness.

Today, Wall Pilates continues to evolve and adapt, with instructors and practitioners alike exploring innovative ways to integrate the wall into their practice. From wall-mounted apparatus to portable straps and resistance bands, the possibilities are endless, offering endless opportunities for exploration and discovery.

As we reflect on the origins and history of Wall Pilates, we are reminded of its enduring legacy as a transformative practice that empowers women to unleash their full potential and embrace a life of strength, balance, and vitality.

Benefits of Wall Pilates

As we venture deeper into the transformative potential of Wall Pilates, let's explore the myriad benefits that await those who embrace this dynamic practice with open arms and open hearts.

Physical Benefits

Wall Pilates is a full-body workout that targets every muscle group with precision and intention. By leveraging the support and resistance of the wall, practitioners engage in a series of controlled movements designed to sculpt lean muscles, improve flexibility, and enhance overall strength. Whether you're a seasoned athlete or a newcomer to the world of fitness, Wall Pilates offers a gentle yet effective way to tone and tighten your body from head to toe.

One of the most noticeable advantages of Wall Pilates is improved posture. As we spend more time hunched over computers and smartphones, our posture can suffer, leading to aches, pains, and imbalances. Wall Pilates helps to counteract these effects by strengthening the core muscles that support the spine and promoting proper alignment throughout the body. With each mindful movement, practitioners learn to stand taller, with shoulders back and head held high—a subtle yet powerful transformation that radiates confidence and poise.

Flexibility is another key component of the Wall Pilates experience. Practitioners gradually expand their range of motion and alleviate tension within the muscles and joints through a sequence of dynamic stretches and lengthening exercises. Whether you're reaching for the sky in a standing stretch or folding forward in a seated position, each movement encourages greater flexibility and freedom of movement, allowing you to move through life with ease and grace.

In addition to improving posture and flexibility, Wall Pilates also helps to build strength from the inside out. By engaging the deep core muscles that stabilize the spine and pelvis, practitioners develop a strong foundation upon which to build greater strength and stability. With each controlled movement, muscles are challenged and refined, resulting in a lean, toned physique that exudes confidence and vitality.

Mental Benefits

Beyond the physical benefits, Wall Pilates also offers a wealth of mental and emotional rewards. As practitioners focus their attention inward and connect with the rhythm of their breath, they enter a state of mindfulness that promotes relaxation and stress relief. With each inhale, tension melts away; with each breathe out, a sense of calm washes over the body and mind. In this way, Wall Pilates serves as a moving meditation—a sanctuary where practitioners can escape the chaos of daily life and find peace within.

In addition to promoting relaxation and stress relief, Wall Pilates also fosters a greater sense of self-awareness and body confidence. As practitioners become attuned to the subtle nuances of their movements, they learn to trust their bodies and honor their unique strengths and limitations. With each session, they develop a deeper understanding of their physical capabilities and cultivate a sense of appreciation for all that their bodies can do.

Furthermore, Wall Pilates can also serve as a powerful tool for mental and emotional healing. Whether you're dealing with chronic pain, recovering from injury, or simply seeking solace from the pressures of modern life, Wall Pilates offers a safe and supportive environment in which to explore and release pent-up emotions. As practitioners move through each exercise with intention and care, they create space for healing and transformation, allowing them to emerge stronger, more resilient, and more connected to their inner selves.

Overall Well-being

As we journey through the world of Wall Pilates, it's important to remember that true well-being encompasses more than just physical fitness—it's about nurturing the body, mind, and spirit in harmony. By embracing the principles of control, concentration, precision, and breath, Wall Pilates promotes health and well-being through the use of an integrated strategy that transcends the boundaries of the studio. Incorporating Wall Pilates into your daily regimen not only enhances your physical fitness but also nurtures mental clarity, emotional resilience, and overall quality of life.

Whether you're seeking to alleviate chronic pain, boost your energy levels, or simply find moments of peace amidst the chaos of daily life, Wall Pilates offers a path to greater health, happiness, and vitality.

Fundamental Principles

Within the practice of Wall Pilates, six foundational principles serve as guiding lights, illuminating the path to physical mastery and inner harmony. Each principle represents a pillar upon which the practice is built, weaving together the threads of control, concentration, precision, and breath into a tapestry of holistic well-being.

1. Control

Control lies at the heart of Wall Pilates, serving as the cornerstone of every movement and gesture. In this practice, control transcends mere physical mastery—it embodies a deep sense of awareness and intentionality that permeates every aspect of one's being. From the subtle engagement of core muscles to the graceful extension of limbs, practitioners cultivate an innate sense of control over their bodies, fostering strength, stability, and resilience.

Through precise, deliberate movements, individuals learn to harness the power of control to sculpt lean muscles, improve posture, and prevent injury. With each exercise, they navigate the delicate balance between effort and ease, finding strength in stillness and grace in motion. As control becomes second nature, practitioners discover a newfound sense of agency over their bodies and minds, empowering them to navigate life's challenges with confidence and poise.

2. Concentration

In the fast-paced rhythm of modern life, the ability to focus and concentrate is a precious commodity—a skill honed to perfection within the realm of Wall Pilates. As practitioners engage in each exercise with unwavering attention and presence, they cultivate a profound sense of mindfulness that extends far beyond the confines of the mat.

Concentration becomes a gateway to deeper self-awareness, allowing individuals to quiet the noise of the external world and turn inward, where true transformation begins. With each breath, each movement, practitioners immerse themselves fully in the present moment, savoring the sensation of muscles engaging, joints aligning, and breath flowing freely.

Through the practice of concentration, individuals develop mental clarity, heightened awareness, and a profound connection to their bodies. As distractions fade into the background and the mind grows still, they discover a profound sense of inner peace and tranquility—a sanctuary amidst the chaos of daily life.

3. Precision

In the world of Wall Pilates, precision reigns supreme—a commitment to excellence that permeates every aspect of the practice. From the alignment of the spine to the positioning of the feet, practitioners strive for perfection in every movement, knowing that even the slightest adjustment can yield profound results.

Precision is not merely about achieving physical perfection—it is about honoring the body's innate intelligence and respecting its limits. Through attentive observation and meticulous attention to detail, individuals acquire the ability to move gracefully and effortlessly, minimizing the risk of unnecessary strain and injury.

As precision becomes a guiding principle, practitioners discover a newfound sense of connection to their bodies—an awareness of subtle nuances and sensations that had previously gone unnoticed. With each movement, they cultivate a deep sense of trust and respect for their bodies, forging a partnership based on mutual understanding and harmony.

4. Breath

The breath is the life force that animates the body, infusing every movement with vitality and purpose. In Wall Pilates, breath serves as a powerful tool for cultivating presence, awareness, and inner peace. Through mindful breathing techniques, practitioners learn to synchronize breath with movement, creating a seamless flow of energy that nourishes body, mind, and spirit.

With each inhale, practitioners draw in fresh oxygen, replenishing cells and revitalizing muscles. With each breathe out, they release tension, stress, and negativity, clearing the way for renewed vitality and clarity. As breath becomes the anchor that grounds them in the present moment, practitioners discover a profound sense of calm and centeredness—a refuge amidst the chaos of daily life.

5. Fluidity

In the practice of Wall Pilates, fluidity is not merely a physical attribute—it is a state of being, characterized by grace, ease, and effortless movement. Through fluid, flowing sequences, practitioners learn to cultivate a sense of fluidity in both body and mind, transcending the limitations of rigidity and resistance.

Fluidity is about embracing the inherent interconnectedness of all things, surrendering to the natural rhythms of life and allowing energy to flow freely. With each movement, practitioners embody the qualities of water—flexible, adaptable, and infinitely resilient.

As fluidity becomes a guiding principle, practitioners discover a newfound sense of freedom and expansiveness—an openness to possibility and change. With each breath, each movement, they surrender to the currents of life, trusting in the inherent wisdom of the body and the universe.

6. Integration

Wall Pilates is a practice of integration—an invitation to unite body, mind, and spirit in a harmonious dance of movement and stillness. Through seamless integration of breath, movement, and intention, practitioners learn to cultivate a sense of wholeness and balance that transcends the confines of the physical body.

Integration is about recognizing the interconnectedness of all things and honoring the inherent wisdom of the body. It is about listening deeply to the signals and sensations that arise within, trusting in the body's innate intelligence to guide us on the path to health and vitality.

As practitioners integrate the principles of Wall Pilates into their daily lives, they discover a profound sense of alignment and purpose—a deep knowing that they are part of something greater than themselves. With each breath, each movement, they celebrate the miracle of being alive, embracing the journey with open hearts and open minds.

Structure of the Book

Before delving into the intricate details of Wall Pilates exercises and routines, let's take a moment to explore the structure of this book.

1. Practical Advice

Space Preparation:

Before diving into the world of Wall Pilates, it's vital to create a conducive environment for practice. This chapter offers practical advice on setting up your practice space, including choosing the right location, optimizing lighting, and ensuring cleanliness for a focused and energizing session.

Essential Tools:

This section provides guidance on purchasing and using essential tools for Wall Pilates.

Adequate Heating:

Prepare your body for movement with targeted warm-up routines. Discover specific warm-up exercises tailored to prime your body—neck, shoulders, wrists, ankles, and more—ensuring readiness and reducing the risk of injury before delving into your Wall Pilates practice.

Correct Execution of the Exercises:

Unlock the full potential of Wall Pilates with detailed instructions on executing each exercise correctly. Learn about body positioning, breathing techniques, and muscle control to maximize the effectiveness of your practice and achieve optimal results.

Gradual Progression:

Tailor your practice to your skill level and physical condition with guidance on planning a gradual progression. Whether you're a beginner or seasoned practitioner, adapt exercises to suit your needs and steadily advance on your journey with Wall Pilates.

Rest and Recovery:

Recognize the significance of rest and recovery in sustaining a well-rounded practice. Explore effective strategies to integrate ample rest periods and recovery techniques into your routine, aiming to prevent fatigue, optimize performance, and mitigate the risk of injury.

Advice on Consistency:

Stay motivated and committed to your practice with practical tips for maintaining consistency. Explore strategies for integrating Wall Pilates seamlessly into your daily routine, ensuring ongoing progress and sustainable results.

Possible Adaptations:

Navigate physical limitations or specific conditions with tips on adapting exercises to suit your individual needs. Whether you're recovering from an injury or managing a chronic condition, discover modifications that empower you to participate fully in the transformative practice of Wall Pilates.

2. Exercises

Dive into a curated collection of fortyWall Pilates exercises, divided into four targeted groups: Total Body, Core (abdominals and lumbar back), Legs and Buttocks, and Arms and Shoulders. Each exercise is presented with clear and detailed instructions, including beginner and advanced versions, step-by-step guidance, and accompanying images or illustrations to ensure proper execution and understanding.

3. 28-Day Workout (Beginners)

Embark on a transformative 28-day journey with a structured workout plan designed for beginners. Each daily program features a selection of exercises from the beginner level, presented in a table format for easy reference. Start gradually, increasing difficulty and intensity over time, and experience the transformative power of consistent practice.

4. Workout 7 Days (Advanced Level)

Challenge yourself with a seven-day workout plan tailored to the advanced level practitioner. Similar to the 28-day program, each daily workout features a selection of exercises from the advanced level, offering a balanced and dynamic approach to strength, flexibility, and overall well-being.

5. Bonus Workout 7-Day Abdominal Core (Beginner and Advanced)

Strengthen and tone your abdominal core with a bonus seven-day workout plan focused specifically on this vital area. Explore a selection of exercises aimed at targeting the core abdominals and lumbar back, presented in both beginner and advanced versions for comprehensive development and progression.

6. **Bonus Nutritional Tips**

Complement your workout regimen with essential nutritional guidance for optimal health and vitality. Acquire knowledge about the significance of maintaining a balanced diet and explore practical tips for making informed food choices. These practices are designed to not only support your fitness goals but also contribute to enhancing your overall well-being.

7. **Bonus 7 Breathing Exercises**

Harness the power of conscious breathing to enhance your Wall Pilates practice and promote overall well-being. Explore seven breathing exercises designed to improve mood, reduce stress, and optimize performance, complementing your physical efforts with mindfulness and inner balance.

With each page turned, may you feel a spark of inspiration igniting within—a call to action, a whisper of possibility. Embrace this invitation to practice with an open heart and a curious mind, knowing that the journey ahead holds infinite potential for growth and self-discovery. Whether you're a seasoned practitioner or a newcomer to the world of Pilates, let this book be your companion—a trusted ally on the path to vibrant health and unshakeable strength.

Together, let us embark on this journey—one wall, one breath, one movement at a time—unleashing the boundless potential that resides within. Welcome to the transformative world of Wall Pilates—a place where strength knows no bounds and empowerment reigns supreme

Chapter 1:

Practical Advice

In the pursuit of mastering Wall Pilates, preparation and understanding of the environment, tools, and practices are essential. This chapter serves as your comprehensive guide, offering invaluable advice and insights to optimize your Wall Pilates experience and ensure a safe and effective practice. From setting up your practice space to adapting exercises based on individual needs, let us explore each aspect in detail.

Space Preparation

Setting up a conducive space for your Wall Pilates practice is essential for maximizing focus, safety, and effectiveness. This section will focus on the most important factors to take into account and practical tips for preparing your practice area to ensure a transformative and rewarding experience.

Choosing the Location

Selecting the right location for your Wall Pilates practice sets the stage for success. Aim for a spacious area with sufficient room for movement and minimal obstructions. Ideally, choose a quiet and peaceful environment free from distractions, allowing you to fully immerse yourself in the practice and cultivate mindfulness. Consider natural elements such as sunlight and fresh air to enhance your overall well-being and create a harmonious atmosphere for your practice.

Optimizing Lighting

Proper lighting is essential for maintaining clarity and visibility during your Wall Pilates sessions. Aim for a well-lit space with ample natural or artificial light to ensure clear visibility of your surroundings and proper alignment during exercises. Position yourself in a well-illuminated area, avoiding harsh or glaring lights that may cause discomfort or distraction.

Maintaining Cleanliness

Keeping your practice space clean and organized is crucial for promoting a sense of calm, clarity, and focus. Prioritize cleanliness by removing clutter and unnecessary items from your practice area, creating a clean and uncluttered environment conducive to movement and mindfulness. Regularly clean and sanitize your equipment, props, and surfaces to ensure hygiene and prevent the buildup of dust and allergens.

Creating Ambiance

Enhance the ambiance of your practice space to promote relaxation, inspiration, and positive energy. Consider incorporating elements such as soothing music, aromatherapy, and inspiring visuals to create a multi-sensory experience that nourishes the body, mind, and spirit. Experiment with a variety of odors, sounds, and visual clues to determine what connects with you and makes your practice more effective.

Personalizing Your Space

Make your practice space uniquely yours by infusing it with elements that reflect your personality, preferences, and intentions. Personalize your space with meaningful decorations, inspiring quotes, or items that hold special significance to you. Consider creating a dedicated altar or meditation corner where you can set intentions, express gratitude, and connect with your inner self before and after your Wall Pilates practice.

Setting Intentions

Before each practice session, take a moment to set intentions for your practice, focusing on what you hope to cultivate and achieve. Whether it's strength, flexibility, balance, or inner peace, clarify your intentions and visualize yourself embodying them throughout your practice. Consider dedicating a few moments of quiet reflection or meditation to center yourself and connect with your intentions before beginning your Wall Pilates practice.

Prepare Your Tools

In addition to setting up your space, preparing the necessary tools for your Wall Pilates practice is essential for a safe and effective workout. One of the primary tools you'll need is a high-quality Pilates mat to provide cushioning and support for your body during floor exercises. Here are some tips for selecting and preparing your mat: invest in a Pilates mat that offers adequate thickness (usually around 10-15mm) to cushion your body and joints during exercises. Look for a non-slip surface to prevent sliding, ensuring stability and safety throughout your practice.

Purchase, if you don't already own them, snug-fitting yoga or Pilates attire to be as comfortable as possible. I suggest using the attire only when exercising to prioritize your practice more.

Adequate Heating

Before delving into the dynamic movements of Wall Pilates, it's essential to adequately prepare your body for the challenges ahead. Adequate heating not only helps to prevent injury but also primes your muscles, joints, and connective tissues for optimal performance and flexibility.

Importance of Warm-Up

A proper warm-up is crucial for increasing blood flow, improving flexibility, and enhancing neuromuscular activation before engaging in strenuous physical activity. By gradually increasing heart rate and body temperature, warm-up exercises prepare your body for the demands of Wall Pilates, reducing the risk of injury and ensuring a more effective and enjoyable practice experience. Moreover, warming up contributes to joint lubrication, loosens tight muscles, and enhances range of motion. This facilitates increased freedom and ease of movement during your Pilates session.

Specific Warm-Up Routines

1. **Neck Warm-Up:** Start by softly tilting your head sideways, bringing your ear towards your shoulder, and maintaining this position for a few seconds on each side. Then, proceed to execute gentle circular motions with your head, rotating both clockwise and counterclockwise. This movement aids in alleviating tension and enhancing mobility in the neck muscles.

2. **Shoulder Warm-Up:** Start by rolling your shoulders forward in slow, controlled circles, gradually increasing the range of motion with each repetition. Then, reverse the direction and roll your shoulders backward, focusing on opening up the chest and releasing tension in the shoulder muscles. Finally, perform shoulder shrugs, lifting your shoulders towards your ears and then relaxing them down, repeating several times to release tension and improve circulation in the shoulders.

3. **Wrist Warm-Up:** The palms of your hands ought to be facing down when you extend your arms straight in front of you at shoulder height. Begin by gently flexing and extending your wrists, moving your hands up and down in a controlled motion. Then, rotate your wrists in circles, alternating between clockwise and counterclockwise rotations to improve flexibility and circulation in the wrists and forearms.

4. **Ankle Warm-Up:** Sit or stand with your feet flat on the floor, hip-width apart. Begin by flexing and pointing your toes, alternating between dorsiflexion and plantarflexion to warm up the ankle joints and calf muscles. Then, rotate your ankles in circles, moving in

both clockwise and counterclockwise directions to improve mobility and circulation in the ankles and lower legs.

5. **Spinal Warm-Up:** Start in a seated or standing position with your spine tall and straight. Begin by gently twisting your torso to one side, reaching one arm across your body and placing the opposite hand on the outside of the thigh or knee. Hold the twist for a few breaths, then return to center and repeat on the other side. This gentle spinal twist helps to warm up the muscles along the spine and improve spinal mobility for Wall Pilates practice.

6. **Hip Warm-Up:** Stand with your feet hip-width apart and hands on your hips. Begin by gently swaying your hips from side to side, shifting your weight from one foot to the other to loosen up the hip joints and improve circulation in the hip muscles. Then, perform hip circles, moving your hips in a circular motion, alternating between clockwise and counterclockwise rotations to warm up the hip joints and increase mobility in the pelvis.

Correct Execution of the Exercises

In Wall Pilates, mastering correct execution of the exercises is paramount to reaping the full advantages of this transformative practice. Each movement is carefully designed to engage specific muscles, improve flexibility, and enhance overall body awareness.

Body Position

At the heart of correct exercise execution lies impeccable body position. Before initiating any movement, establish a strong foundation by standing tall with feet hip-width apart, shoulders relaxed, and spine elongated. Engage the core muscles by drawing the navel towards the spine and gently tucking the tailbone under to stabilize the pelvis. Maintain a neutral alignment of the spine, with the head stacked directly over the shoulders and the pelvis in a neutral position.

Throughout each exercise, pay close attention to your body's alignment and posture. Avoid overarching or rounding the spine, and strive to keep the body in a straight line from head to heels. Engage the muscles of the upper back and shoulders to maintain an open chest and proud posture, promoting proper alignment and maximizing the effectiveness of each movement.

Breathing Techniques

Breath is the life force that sustains us, and in Wall Pilates, it serves as the rhythm that guides our movements. Practice diaphragmatic breathing, inhaling deeply through the nose to expand the ribcage and belly, and exhaling fully through the mouth to draw the navel towards the spine and engage the core muscles. Coordinate your breath with each movement by inhaling to prepare and exhaling to initiate the movement. Let your breath flow naturally and effortlessly throughout your practice, creating a harmonious connection between breath and movement.

Conscious breathing not only oxygenates the muscles and enhances circulation but also promotes relaxation and mindfulness, allowing you to fully immerse yourself in the present moment and connect with the subtle nuances of each movement. Cultivate a steady, rhythmic breath pattern that supports and sustains you as you move through your Wall Pilates practice, harnessing the power of breath to optimize your performance and deepen your mind-body connection.

Muscle Control

The hallmark of a skilled Wall Pilates practitioner lies in their ability to harness the power of muscle control. Focus on engaging the deep stabilizing muscles of the core, including the transverse abdominis, pelvic floor, and multifidus, to support and stabilize the spine and pelvis throughout each movement. Maintain a sense of dynamic tension in the muscles, avoiding excessive tension or gripping, and focus on initiating movement from the core while maintaining stability in the surrounding muscles and joints.

Mindful muscle activation is essential for maximizing the effectiveness of Wall Pilates exercises and minimizing the risk of injury. Concentrate on contracting and releasing the muscles with precision and control, paying attention to the subtle sensations and feedback from your body. Visualize the muscles engaging and lengthening with each movement, cultivating a deep awareness and connection with your body as you move through your Pilates practice.

Gradual Progression

As you begin your practice, it's essential to embrace the concept of gradual progression—a principle that will guide you on your path to mastery and help you unlock your full potential. Here, we'll explore the importance of gradual progression in your practice, offering advice on how to plan and adapt exercises based on individual skill levels and physical conditions.

1. Assessing Your Starting Point

Before diving into Wall Pilates, take time to assess your current skill level, strength, flexibility, and overall physical condition. Be honest with yourself about your abilities and limitations, and use this assessment to establish a baseline for your practice. Start with foundational exercises and movements that align with your current capabilities, allowing room for growth and improvement over time.

2. Setting Realistic Goals

Once you have assessed your starting point, set realistic and achievable goals for your Wall Pilates practice. Whether it's improving core strength, enhancing flexibility, or alleviating back pain, define specific goals that are meaningful to you and align with your motivations for practicing Pilates. Break down overarching goals into smaller, measurable milestones, and take the time to celebrate your progress as you strive towards their accomplishment.

3. Planning Your Progression

Design a structured progression plan that gradually increases the intensity, duration, and complexity of your Wall Pilates workouts. Start with basic exercises and gradually incorporate more challenging variations and sequences as you build strength, flexibility, and confidence. Listen to your body's feedback and adjust the pace of progression accordingly, allowing for periods of rest and recovery as needed to prevent burnout and injury.

4. Adapting Exercises for Individual Needs

Acknowledge that each individual's body is distinct, understanding that what proves effective for one person may not yield the same results for another. Adapt exercises based on individual skill levels, physical conditions, and limitations to ensure a safe and effective practice experience. Modify exercises as needed by using props, adjusting range of motion, or reducing resistance to accommodate injuries, mobility issues, or specific conditions. Consult with a qualified Pilates instructor or healthcare professional for personalized guidance and recommendations tailored to your individual needs.

5. Embracing Variation and Challenge

Keep your Wall Pilates practice engaging and dynamic by incorporating variation and challenge into your workouts. Experiment with different exercises, props, and sequences to target different muscle groups and movement patterns, stimulating continuous growth and improvement. Challenge yourself to try new movements and progressions, stepping outside your comfort zone to expand your repertoire and enhance your skills. Embrace the journey of exploration and discovery, and let each workout be an opportunity for growth and self-discovery.

6. Listening to Your Body

Above all, listen to your body and honor its signals and needs throughout your Wall Pilates practice. Pay attention to signs of fatigue, discomfort, or pain, and adjust your intensity or modify your exercises accordingly. Allow yourself time to rest and recover between workouts, prioritizing self-care practices such as stretching, foam rolling, and relaxation techniques to support your body's natural healing processes. Trust in your body's wisdom and intuition, and cultivate a compassionate and nurturing relationship with yourself as you navigate your Pilates journey.

Rest and Recovery

In the pursuit of mastery in Wall Pilates, it's essential to recognize the importance of rest and recovery in maintaining optimal health and performance. Rest is not only essential for physical recovery but also for mental and emotional rejuvenation. When you engage in intense physical activity such as Wall Pilates, your muscles experience micro-tears and fatigue, which require time to repair and rebuild stronger. Additionally, rest allows your nervous system to recalibrate, your energy stores to replenish, and your mind to decompress from stress and tension. By prioritizing rest in your Pilates practice, you create the conditions for optimal growth, performance, and overall well-being.

Planning Rest Periods

Incorporate regular rest periods into your Wall Pilates routine to allow your body to recover and adapt to the demands of exercise. Schedule rest days between intense workouts or incorporate active recovery activities such as gentle stretching, walking, or yoga to promote circulation, flexibility, and relaxation. Listen to your body's cues and adjust your training schedule accordingly, allowing for additional rest days or lighter workouts when needed to prevent overtraining and burnout.

Implementing Recovery Strategies

In addition to rest, implementing effective recovery strategies can further support your body's recovery and enhance your performance in Wall Pilates. Incorporate post-workout stretching to alleviate muscle tension and improve flexibility, focusing on areas that feel tight or fatigued. Use foam rolling or self-myofascial release techniques to release knots and trigger points in your muscles, promoting blood flow and reducing soreness. Prioritize hydration and nutrition by fueling your body with nutrient-rich foods and staying adequately hydrated to support muscle repair and replenish energy stores.

Prioritizing Sleep

Quality sleep is a cornerstone of recovery and essential for overall health and well-being. Aim for seven to nine hours of restorative sleep each night to facilitate muscle repair, hormone regulation, and cognitive function. Create a sleep-friendly environment by establishing a consistent bedtime routine, minimizing exposure to screens and electronic devices before bed, and ensuring your sleep environment is dark, quiet, and comfortable. Prioritize sleep as a non-negotiable component of your recovery regimen, and reap the advantages of improved performance, mood, and vitality in your Wall Pilates practice and daily life.

Practicing Stress Management

Embed stress management techniques into your daily schedule to aid recovery and strengthen resilience in the face of life's challenges. Engage in activities such as meditation, deep breathing exercises, or gentle movement practices to promote relaxation and reduce the physiological effects of stress on the body. Cultivate mindfulness and self-awareness, tuning into your body's signals and responding with compassion and kindness. By managing stress effectively, you create a supportive internal environment that fosters healing, balance, and well-being, both on and off the mat.

Honoring Your Body's Wisdom

Above all, honor your body's wisdom and prioritize self-care practices that support your health and vitality. Listen to your body's signals and needs, and respond with kindness, compassion, and respect. Trust in your body's innate ability to heal, restore, and thrive, and cultivate a nurturing relationship with yourself that prioritizes well-being and self-love. By honoring your body's wisdom and nurturing yourself from the inside out, you lay the foundation for a sustainable and fulfilling Pilates practice that supports your long-term health, happiness, and vitality.

Advice on Consistency

Consistency is the key to success in Wall Pilates, as it fosters progress, builds momentum, and cultivates lasting transformation in both body and mind. Here, we'll explore strategies for maintaining a consistent practice over time and incorporating Wall Pilates into your daily routine for maximum impact and benefits.

1. Establishing a Routine

Create a dedicated space and time for your Wall Pilates practice to ensure consistency and commitment. Whether it's a corner of your living room, a local Pilates studio, or an outdoor space, make it a sanctuary for your practice, free from distractions and interruptions. Schedule your Pilates sessions at a consistent time each day or week, integrating them into your daily routine like any other essential activity. By establishing a routine, you cultivate discipline, structure, and accountability, making it easier to prioritize and sustain your Pilates practice over time.

2. Setting Realistic Expectations

Set realistic and achievable expectations for your Pilates practice, taking into account your schedule, lifestyle, and commitments. Be flexible and adaptable, recognizing that some days may be busier or more challenging than others, and adjust your expectations accordingly. Focus on consistency and progress rather than perfection, and celebrate small victories and milestones along the way. By setting realistic expectations, you create a positive and empowering mindset that supports your long-term success and satisfaction in your Pilates journey.

3. Finding Motivation and Inspiration

Stay motivated and inspired in your Pilates practice by connecting with your inner motivation and tapping into external sources of inspiration. Reflect on your reasons for practicing Pilates, whether it's to improve your health, alleviate pain, enhance performance, or simply feel good in your body. Draw inspiration from Pilates instructors, fellow practitioners, and online communities, surrounding yourself with like-minded individuals who share your passion and enthusiasm for Pilates. Set goals, track your progress, and reward yourself for your achievements, fueling your motivation and commitment to your practice.

4. Cultivating Mindfulness and Presence

Cultivate mindfulness and presence in your Pilates practice by bringing awareness to the present moment and tuning into your body's sensations, thoughts, and emotions. Practice mindful breathing techniques to ground yourself and center your attention, allowing distractions to fade away as you immerse yourself fully in the present experience. Let go of judgment and comparison, and embrace a spirit of curiosity, exploration, and self-discovery in your practice. By cultivating mindfulness and presence, you deepen your connection to yourself and your practice, enhancing the quality and effectiveness of your Pilates experience.

5. Embracing Variety and Exploration

Keep your Pilates practice fresh and exciting by embracing variety and exploration in your workouts. Experiment with different exercises, props, and class formats to challenge your body and mind in new ways and prevent boredom or plateaus. Explore different styles of Pilates, such as mat Pilates, reformer Pilates, or aerial Pilates, to broaden your repertoire and expand your skills. Incorporate cross-training activities such as yoga, dance, or strength training to complement your Pilates practice and enhance overall fitness and performance. Embrace the spirit of exploration and curiosity, and let each Pilates session be an opportunity for growth, learning, and self-expression.

6. Prioritizing Self-Care and Recovery

Prioritize self-care and recovery as essential components of your Pilates practice, allowing time for rest, relaxation, and rejuvenation to support your overall well-being. Listen to your body's signals and needs, and honor them with kindness and compassion, incorporating rest days, active recovery activities, and stress management techniques into your routine. Nourish your body with nutritious foods, stay hydrated, and prioritize quality sleep to support optimal health and vitality. By prioritizing self-care and recovery, you create a supportive and sustainable foundation for your Pilates practice, allowing you to thrive both on and off the mat.

Possible Adaptations

In the practice of Wall Pilates, it's essential to recognize that one size does not fit all, and flexibility and adaptability are key to meeting the diverse needs of practitioners. In this section, we'll explore tips and strategies for adapting exercises to accommodate physical limitations, injuries, or specific conditions, ensuring an inclusive and accessible practice experience for all.

1. **Listen to Your Body**: The first and most important step in adapting exercises is to listen to your body's signals and respond with kindness, compassion, and respect. Pay attention to any discomfort, pain, or limitations you may experience during exercise, and adjust your movements accordingly to prevent exacerbating existing issues or causing new injuries. Trust in your body's wisdom and intuition, and honor its unique needs and limitations with patience and understanding.

2. **Modify Range of Motion**: If you have limited mobility or flexibility in certain areas of your body, consider modifying the range of motion in exercises to accommodate your individual needs. Reduce the range of motion or intensity of movements to a level that feels comfortable and safe for your body, gradually increasing as your flexibility and strength improve over time. Focus on performing movements with precision and control, prioritizing quality over quantity to maximize the advantages of each exercise.

3. **Use Props for Support**: Utilize props such as blocks, straps, or cushions to provide additional support and stability during exercises, especially if you have balance issues or joint instability. Props can help modify exercises to make them more accessible and comfortable for individuals with physical limitations or injuries, allowing you to safely engage in Pilates practice without compromising your well-being. Experiment with different props and modifications to find what works best for your body and enhances your practice experience.

4. **Choose Alternative Exercises**: If certain exercises are contraindicated or uncomfortable for your body, choose alternative exercises that target the same muscle groups or movement patterns without exacerbating your condition. Work with a qualified Pilates instructor or healthcare professional to identify suitable alternatives and modifications tailored to your individual needs and goals. Focus on selecting exercises that align with your abilities and limitations, allowing you to participate fully in your Pilates practice with confidence and ease.

5. **Focus on Core Stability**: Regardless of your physical condition or limitations, prioritize core stability and alignment in your Pilates practice to support overall strength, balance, and posture. Emphasize exercises that target the deep stabilizing muscles of the core, including the transverse abdominis, pelvic floor, and multifidus, to provide support and stability to your spine and pelvis. Keeping correct alignment and remaining engaged throughout each exercise should be your primary focus, adapting as needed to accommodate your individual needs and limitations.

6. **Seek Professional Guidance**: If you're unsure how to adapt exercises or modify your Pilates practice to suit your individual needs, seek guidance from a qualified Pilates instructor or healthcare professional. A knowledgeable instructor can provide personalized recommendations, modifications, and adaptations tailored to your specific condition or limitations, ensuring a safe and effective practice experience. Communicate openly with your instructor about any concerns or challenges you may have, and work together to form a practice plan that meets your needs and supports your goals.

Chapter 2

Exercises

TOTAL BODY   **1 Wall Roll Downs**

Affected area: Total body.

Objectives of the Exercise: The Wall Roll Downs exercise is designed to improve flexibility, mobility, and core strength while providing a gentle stretch to the spine and hamstrings. This exercise helps to increase body awareness, improve posture, and enhance overall movement efficiency.

Step-by-Step Instructions:

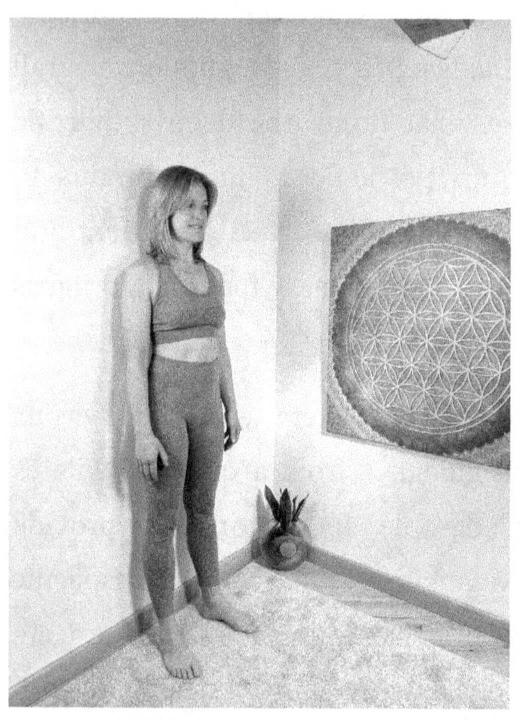

1. **Starting Position:** Stand with your feet hip-width apart, positioned a few inches away from the wall to maintain stability. Ensure your spine is in a neutral position, shoulders relaxed, and arms hanging naturally by your sides.

2. **Breathing:** Breathe in deeply, expanding your ribcage and filling your lungs with air. Controlled breathing plays a vital role in sustaining balance and concentration during the exercise.

3. **Initiate the Descent:** As you breathe out, softly tuck your chin toward your chest to elongate the back of your neck. Begin the descent by slowly rolling your spine downward, segment by segment, starting from the top of your head.

4. **Spinal Roll Down:** Continue the controlled motion as you articulate through each vertebra, moving towards the wall. Allow your arms to hang naturally as you reach towards the wall with your fingertips. Maintain engagement in your core muscles to support your spine throughout the movement.

5. **Lowered Position:** Upon reaching the lowered position where your fingertips make contact with the wall, take a moment to inhale deeply. Use this inhalation to deepen the stretch along your spine and increase your bodily awareness of the position.

6. **Initiate the Ascent:** Exhale gradually as you begin the ascent, rolling back up towards the starting position. Focus on aligning each vertebra as you sequentially stack your spine back into an upright position. Keep your core muscles engaged to support your spine and maintain proper posture.

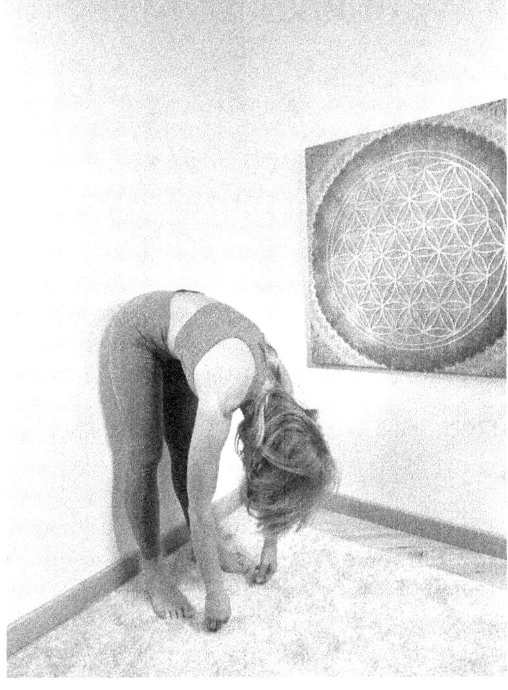

7. **Repetitions:** Aim for 5 to 8 controlled repetitions of the Wall Roll Downs. Focus on maintaining a steady pace throughout each repetition to prevent strain and minimize the risk of injury.

Warnings and Contraindications:

- Individuals with pre-existing back or neck conditions, like herniated discs or spinal instability, should exercise caution when engaging in this exercise. Adjust the range of motion or intensity as necessary to accommodate any physical limitations or discomfort.

Advanced Version:

- **Walk-Out Inchworm:** As you become stronger and more flexible, add variety to the Wall Roll Downs by integrating a walk-out inchworm. After reaching the lowered position with your fingertips on the wall, walk your hands forward along the floor until you achieve a plank position. From the plank position, step one foot up next to the front palm for a lunge stretch, then repeat on the opposite side. You should go back into the plank posture and then walk your hands back over your feet until you are standing again, feeling your core contract as you lift back up. Introducing this modification incorporates dynamic movement, intensifying the challenge on your core muscles and flexibility.

2 Wall Pike

Affected area: Total body, with a focus on core muscles, shoulders, and hamstrings

Objectives of the Exercise: The Wall Pike exercise is a challenging movement that primarily targets the abdominal muscles while also engaging the shoulders, arms, and lower back. This exercise aims to improve core strength, stability, and overall body control. Additionally, it helps enhance flexibility in the hamstrings and hips.

Step-by-Step Instructions:

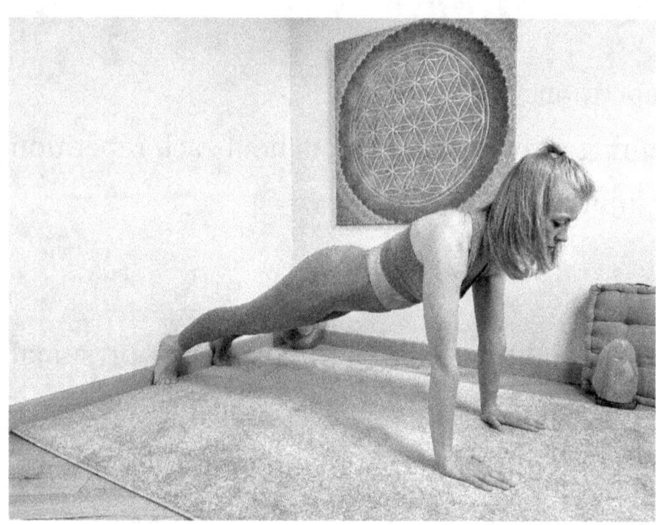

1. **Starting Position:** Begin by assuming a push-up position facing away from the wall, by placing your hands on the floor shoulder-width apart and your feet against the wall, you should be in this position. A straight line should be formed by your body from your head to your heels, and your arms ought to stretch to their fullest, most extended position.

2. **Breathing:** Breathe in deeply through your nose to prepare for the movement.

3. **Initiate the Pike:** Exhale gradually as you engage your core muscles then lift your hips upward toward the ceiling, forming an inverted V shape with your body. Simultaneously, walk your feet up the wall as you pike your hips higher.

4. **Hip Height:** Continue lifting your hips until your body forms an upside-down "V" position, with your torso perpendicular to the floor and your arms and legs straight. Keep your head between your arms, and aim to bring your hips as high as possible while maintaining control.

5. **Hold and Breathing:** Hold the pike position for a moment, maintaining tension in your core muscles and focusing on your breath. Take short, controlled breaths to sustain your balance and stability.

6. **Lowering Down:** Breathe in deeply as you slowly lower your hips back down to the starting push-up position, returning to the straight-line position with your body parallel to the floor.

7. **Repetitions:** Aim to complete 8-10 repetitions of the Wall Pike, focusing on quality over quantity and maintaining proper form throughout each repetition.

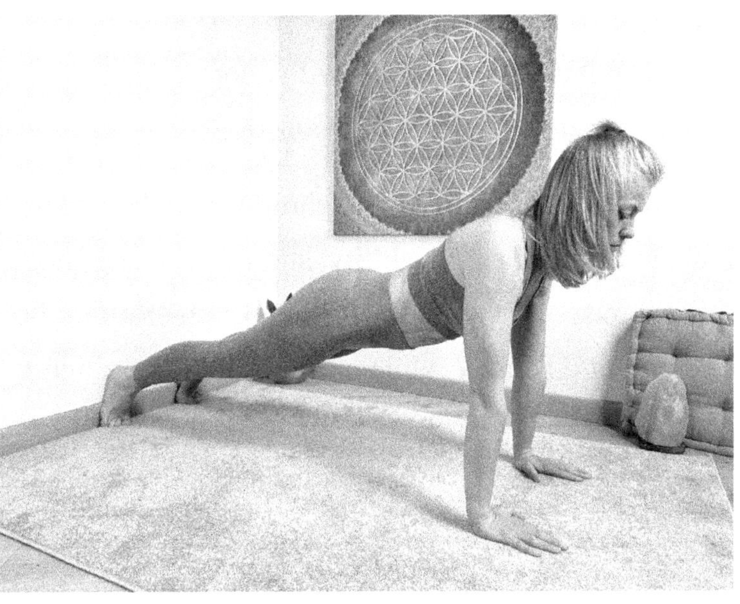

Warnings and Contraindications:

- Avoid overarching your lower back or allowing your hips to sag during the Wall Pike exercise. Focus on maintaining a straight line from your head to your heels throughout the movement to prevent strain on your lower back.
- Individuals with wrist, shoulder, or back issues, such as carpal tunnel syndrome or rotator cuff injuries, should use caution when performing this exercise. Adjust the range of motion or intensity according to your physical limitations or discomfort to ensure a more accommodating and comfortable experience.

Advanced Version:

- **Single-Leg Variation:** Lift one leg off the wall as you pike your hips upward, balancing on the other leg. Hold the single-leg pike position for a few seconds before returning to the starting position. Alternate legs for each repetition to improve balance and stability while increasing the challenge on your core muscles.

3 Wall Walk

Affected Area: Total body, with a focus on core stability, shoulder strength, and coordination.

Objectives of the Exercise: The Wall Walk exercise is a dynamic movement that engages multiple muscle groups throughout the body, including the shoulders, arms, core, and legs. The improvement of core stability, shoulder strength, and overall body control are the key goals of this exercise. By gradually walking the feet up and down the wall, this exercise challenges both strength and balance while promoting proper alignment and posture.

Step-by-Step Instructions:

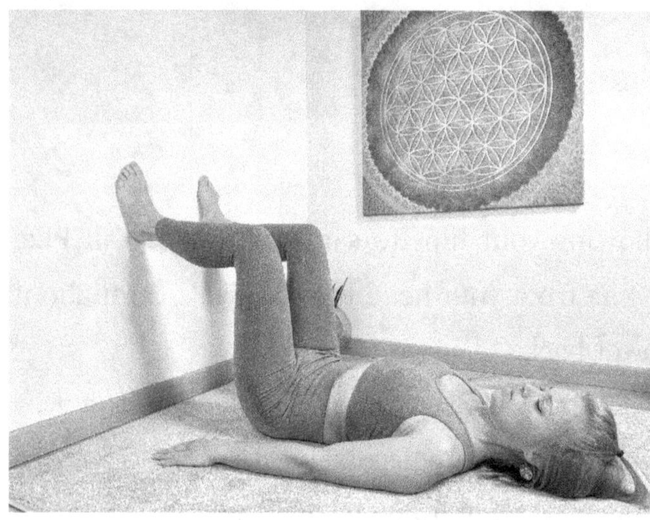

1. **Starting Position:** Begin by lying flat on your back on the floor with your arms comfortably resting at your sides. Bend your knees and place your feet against the wall, ensuring your shins are parallel to the floor. Your hips and knees should be flexed to approximately 90 degrees.

2. **Initiate the Movement:** Gradually initiate the movement by walking your feet up the wall, one step at a time. Maintain relaxed arms by your sides while engaging your core muscles to ensure stability throughout the exercise. Focus on pressing through your heels and keeping your weight evenly distributed on both feet.

3. **Diagonal Position:** Lift your hips and simultaneously walk up the wall until both legs are fully extended; maintain the position for 5 seconds.

4. **Return to Starting Position:** To return to the starting position, carefully and steadily walk your feet back down the wall. Ensure a controlled descent, lowering your hips and

knees while keeping your core engaged to avoid arching or sagging in the lower back. Ensure your movements are deliberate and slow to uphold control and stability.

5. **Complete the Repetition:** Keep walking your feet down the wall until you return to the initial lying position on the floor. Ensure your arms are still resting comfortably at your sides and your feet remain against the wall. This completes one repetition of the Wall Walk exercise.

6. **Repetitions and Sets:** Aim to perform 2-3 sets of 5-10 Wall Walks, adjusting the number of repetitions based on your individual strength and fitness level. Allow for a brief rest period between sets to maintain form and prevent fatigue-related errors.

Warnings and Contraindications:

- Avoid overarching or sagging in the lower back during the Wall Walk exercise. Remember to keep your spine in a neutral position and activate your core muscles to support your lower back throughout the movement.
- Individuals with shoulder impingement or instability should use caution when performing this exercise and may need to modify the range of motion or intensity to avoid exacerbating their condition.

Advanced Version:

- **Single-leg candlestick pose:** Once you reach the diagonal position, support your hips with your hands, pointing your elbows to the ground. Lift your right leg away from the wall for 2 or 3 seconds, then bring it back to the wall and perform the same movement with the left leg. Return gently to the starting position while in a vertical position.

4 Triceps Push-Up With Side Leg Lift

Affected Area: Total body, with a focus on triceps, core stability, and hip abduction.

Objectives of the Exercise: The Triceps Push-Up With Side Leg Lift is designed to target the triceps, core, and lower body simultaneously. This dynamic move not only strengthens and tones the back of your arms but also engages the core muscles and challenges balance and stability. By incorporating the wall for support and resistance, this exercise offers a comprehensive workout, enhancing upper body strength and overall body control.

Step-by-Step Instructions:

1. **Starting Position:** Stand perpendicular to the wall with your left side facing it, ensuring your feet are together. Keep your body in a straight line from head to heels.

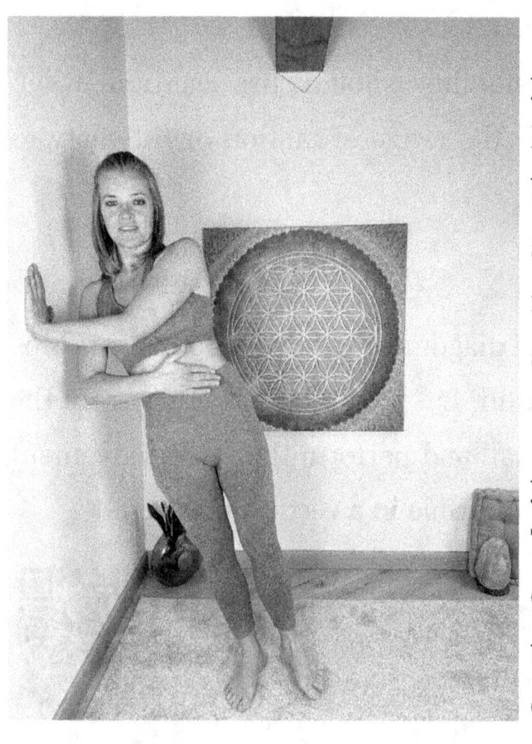

2. **Arm Placement:** Extend your left arm across your chest, placing your palm firmly on the wall. Maintain a distance where you can straighten your elbow but still press into the wall comfortably. Increasing your stability can be accomplished by either crossing your right arm over your chest or wrapping it over your stomach.

3. **Adjustment for Difficulty:** Gradually walk your feet away from the wall to create an inclined angle. The further your feet are from the wall, the more challenging the exercise becomes. Discover a distance that pushes your limits while enabling you to uphold correct form during the exercise.

4. **Initiate the Movement:** Begin the movement by bending your left arm, allowing your torso to lean toward the wall. Keep your elbows close to your body to emphasize the activation of the triceps muscles.

5. **Push Away from the Wall:** Activate your triceps as you push away from the wall, straightening your elbow to return to the initial position. Concentrate on sustaining control and stability throughout the entirety of the movement.

6. **Leg Lift:** Simultaneously, extend your left knee and flex your foot, lifting your left leg to approximately knee height. It is important to engage your core muscles in order to maintain your pelvis and prevent your lower back from arching.

7. **Controlled Lowering:** Lower your left leg without letting it touch the ground. Keep tension in the muscles of your core and hip throughout the movement to control the descent of your leg.

8. **Repetitions:** Complete 10 repetitions of this sequence, maintaining proper form and control throughout. Prioritize precision and control over the number of repetitions, focusing on executing each movement with quality.

9. **Switch Sides:** Once you have completed the number of reps, switch sides and repeat the exercise, facing the opposite direction to target the other arm and leg.

Warnings and Contraindications:

- Avoid overarching or rounding your lower back during the Triceps Push-Up With Side Leg Lift exercise. Focus on maintaining a neutral spine alignment and engaging your core muscles to support your lower back and pelvis.
- Individuals with shoulder injuries, wrist injuries, or any other medical conditions affecting the upper body should use caution when performing this exercise and may need to modify the range of motion or intensity to avoid exacerbating their condition.

Advanced Version:

- **Plyometric Variation:** After completing the triceps push-up, explosively push away from the wall and perform a dynamic side leg lift, aiming to lift your leg as high as possible. This plyometric variation increases power and explosiveness while also challenging your coordination and balance. Ensure that you have mastered the basic exercise before attempting the plyometric variation to decrease the danger of injury.

5 Wall Sit with Arm Raises

Affected Area: Total body, with a focus on arms and shoulders, legs, and core.

Objectives of the Exercise: Offering a full workout for the whole body, the Wall Sit with Arm Raises targets many muscle groups concurrently, making it an ideal strength training exercise. This exercise targets the legs and buttocks for strength and endurance while also working the arms and shoulders through overhead arm raises. In addition, the core muscles are engaged to maintain stability and proper posture throughout the movement.

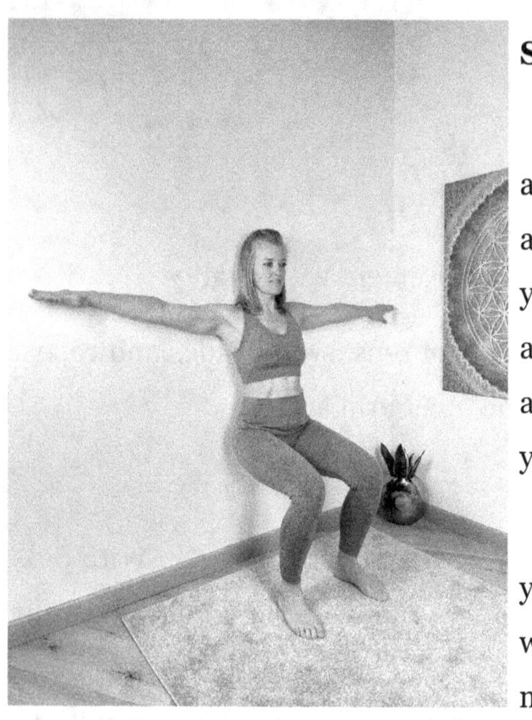

Step-by-Step Instructions:

1. **Starting Position:** Stand with your back against a wall and your feet shoulder-width apart, about two feet away from the wall. As you slide down the wall, lower your body into a seated position and bring your thighs to a position where they are parallel to the floor. In order to achieve a 90-degree angle, you should make sure that your knees are positioned directly above your ankles.

2. **Arm Position:** To perform this exercise, extend your arms straight out to the sides at shoulder height, with your palms facing downward. Ensure your elbows maintain a slight bend to prevent them from locking.

3. **Breathing:** Breathe in deeply through your nose, expanding your chest and filling your lungs with air.

4. **Movement:** Exhale slowly through your mouth as you simultaneously raise your arms overhead, bringing them together until they meet directly above your head. Keep your shoulders relaxed and away from your ears as you perform this movement.

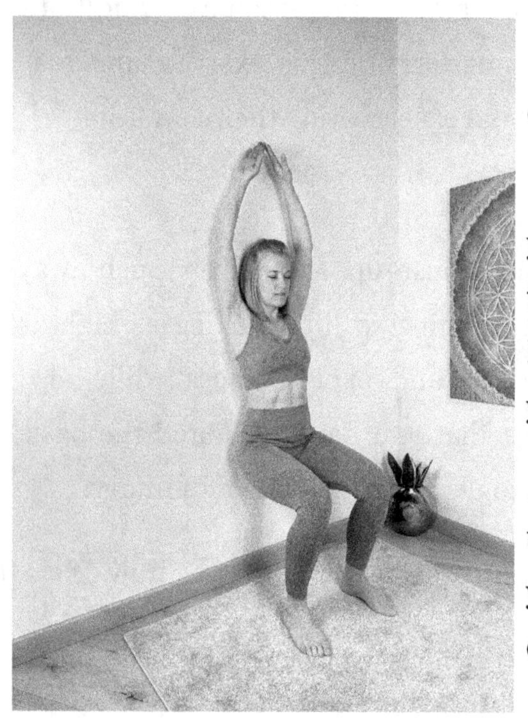

5. **Arm Raises:** Continue lifting your arms overhead until they are fully extended, forming a straight line with your body. Focus on lengthening through your spine and engaging your core muscles to maintain stability.

6. **Hold and Lower:** Hold the raised position for a moment, feeling the stretch in your arms and shoulders. Then, inhale as you slowly lower your arms back to shoulder height, returning to the starting position with control.

7. **Repetitions:** Aim to complete 10-12 repetitions of the Wall Sit with Arm Raises, maintaining the seated position against the wall throughout the exercise.

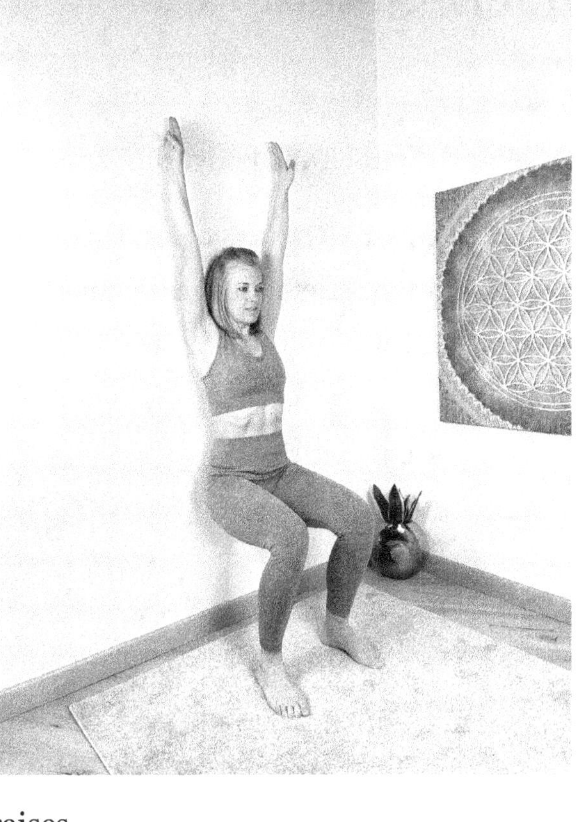

Warnings and Contraindications:

- Avoid holding your breath during the exercise. Remember to breathe continuously and rhythmically, inhaling during the starting position and exhaling during the arm raises.
- Individuals with knee or hip issues, such as arthritis or joint pain, should use caution when performing the Wall Sit with Arm Raises and may need to adjust the depth of the wall sit or the range of motion of the arm raises to avoid exacerbating their condition.

Advanced Version:

- **Pulse Raises:** Instead of lifting your arms overhead in one smooth motion, perform small pulses upward at shoulder height for added muscle burn and endurance. Maintain control and avoid swinging your arms during the pulses to maximize effectiveness.

6 Roll-Up into Bridge

Affected Area: Total body, with a focus on core muscles, glutes, and back.

Objectives of the Exercise: This exercise, known as the Roll-Up into Bridge, is a dynamic movement that stimulates many muscle groups concurrently, making it an excellent choice for giving a full workout for the whole body. Its primary objectives are to improve core strength, flexibility, and spinal mobility while also engaging the glutes and promoting overall body awareness and control.

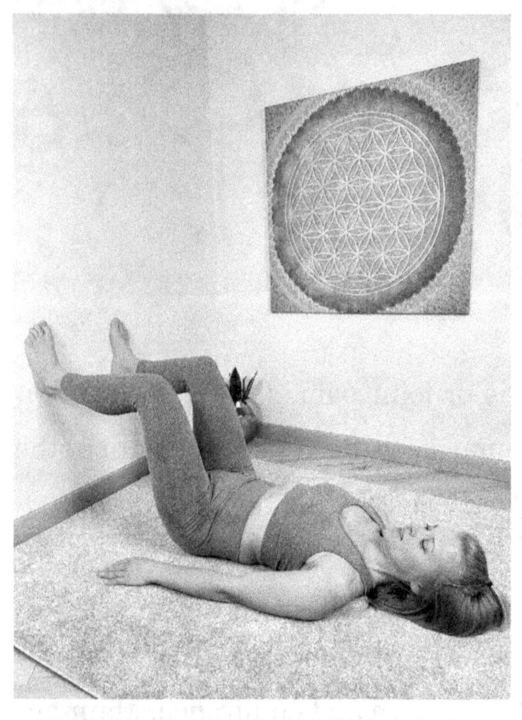

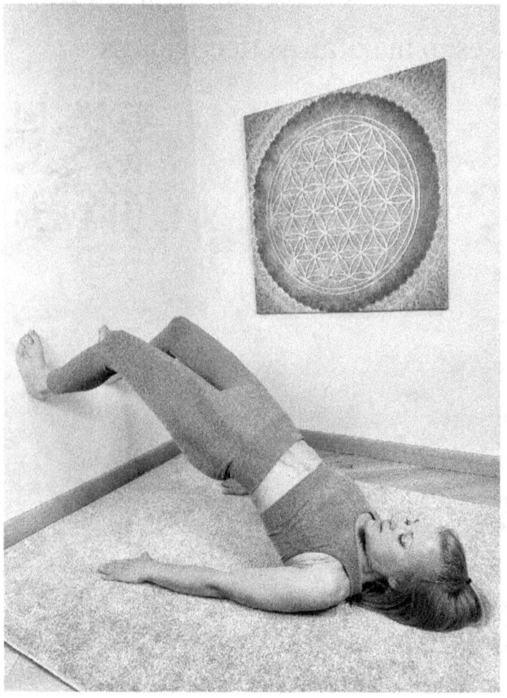

Step-by-Step Instructions:

1. **Starting Position:** Sit facing the wall with your knees bent, ensuring they are positioned about hip-width apart. Begin by rolling down onto your back, maintaining the feet flat against the wall with knees bent at approximately 90 degrees.

2. **Arm Position:** Extend your arms straight in front of you at chest level, with your palms facing down. Engage your core muscles to stabilize your spine and support the movement.

3. **Initiate the Roll-Up:** Tuck your chin toward your chest to initiate the movement, engaging your abdominal muscles. Begin to roll up to a seated position, focusing on lifting one vertebra at a time. Use controlled movements throughout the roll-up, avoiding any jerky or abrupt motions.

4. **Seated Position:** Once you reach a seated position, rest your arms by your sides while maintaining stability. Your spine should be in a neutral position, with your shoulders relaxed and your chest lifted.

5. **Transition to Bridge:** Smoothly transition by drawing your pubic bone toward your belly button, engaging your core muscles. Press your feet into the wall

to activate your glutes and lift your hips into a full bridge position. Ensure your shoulders remain relaxed, and avoid overarching your lower back.

6. **Hold the Bridge:** Once in the bridge position, maintain stability and control by engaging your core muscles and pressing evenly through your feet. Focus on keeping your hips lifted and your spine aligned from shoulders to knees.

7. **Reverse the Movements:** With precision, reverse the movements by scooping your pubic bone toward your belly button, initiating the descent. Slowly lower your back and hips to the floor, one vertebra at a time. Control the descent, allowing each vertebra to touch the ground sequentially.

8. **Repeat:** Repeat the entire sequence for a set of 10 repetitions, maintaining a consistent and controlled pace throughout the movement.

Warnings and Contraindications:

- When performing the Roll-Up into Bridge exercise, be mindful to avoid straining your neck or lower back. Concentrate on activating your core muscles to provide support for your spine and uphold correct alignment throughout the entire motion.
- Individuals with pre-existing back or neck conditions, such as herniated discs or spinal instability, should use caution when performing this exercise and may need to modify the range of motion or intensity to prevent exacerbating their condition.

Advanced Version:

- **Single-Leg Bridge:** Try performing the bridge with one leg lifted off the ground. Elevate one leg straight up towards the ceiling while ensuring the other foot remains firmly pressed against the wall. Maintain the single-leg bridge stance for numerous seconds before reverting to the initial position, then repeat the sequence on the opposite side. This variation increases the challenge on your core muscles and requires greater stability and balance. Alternate between legs for each repetition to ensure balanced muscle engagement and coordination.

7 Single-Leg Bridge with Abduction

Affected Area: Total body, with a focus on core stability, glute strength, and hip mobility.

Objectives of the Exercise: A full workout for the entire body is provided by the Single-Leg Bridge with Abduction exercise, which works many muscle groups concurrently so giving an extensive workout. Its primary objectives are to strengthen the core, glutes, and hip abductors while improving stability, balance, and overall lower body strength.

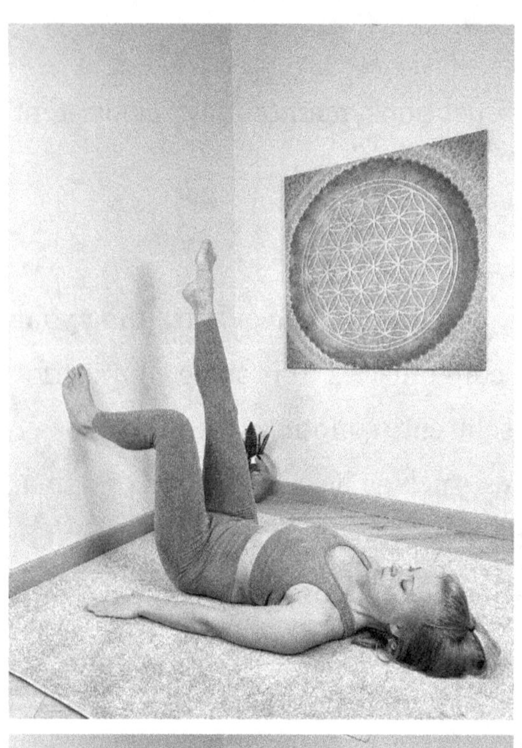

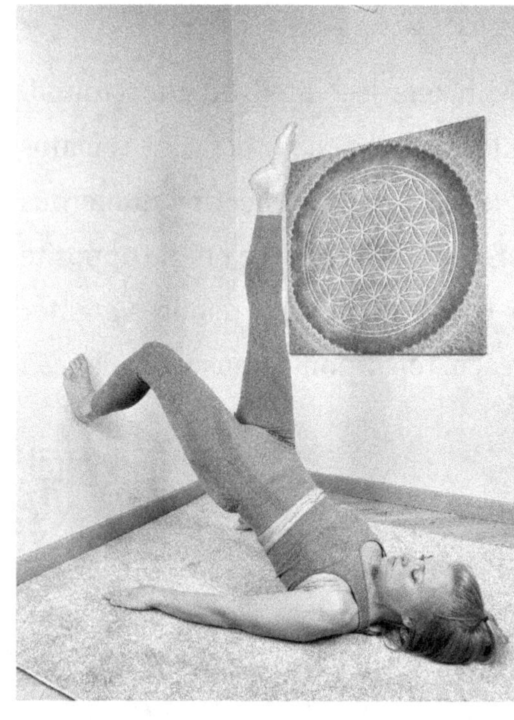

Step-by-Step Instructions:

1. **Starting Position:** Begin by sitting facing the wall with your knees bent, rolling onto your back, and placing your feet flat on the wall. Ensure that your feet are hip-width apart, and your knees are at a 90-degree angle. Keep your arms resting on the ground by your sides, palms facing down.

2. **Positioning the Legs:** Press your left foot against the wall, extending your right knee upward towards the ceiling. Point your toes toward the ceiling to engage the muscles in your right leg.

3. **Activate the Core:** Activate your core muscles by pulling the pubic bone toward your belly button. This action helps to stabilize your pelvis and protect your lower back throughout the movement.

4. **Raise the Hips:** Apply pressure on your left foot to raise your hips off the ground, forming a complete bridge position. Ensure that your pelvis remains level throughout the movement, avoiding any tilting or twisting.

5. **Perform Abduction:** Once in the bridge position, move your right leg outward (abduct it) away from your body's midline. Focus on engaging the muscles

on the outside of your hip to lift your leg while keeping your right hip stable. Avoid allowing your pelvis to drop or rotate during this movement.

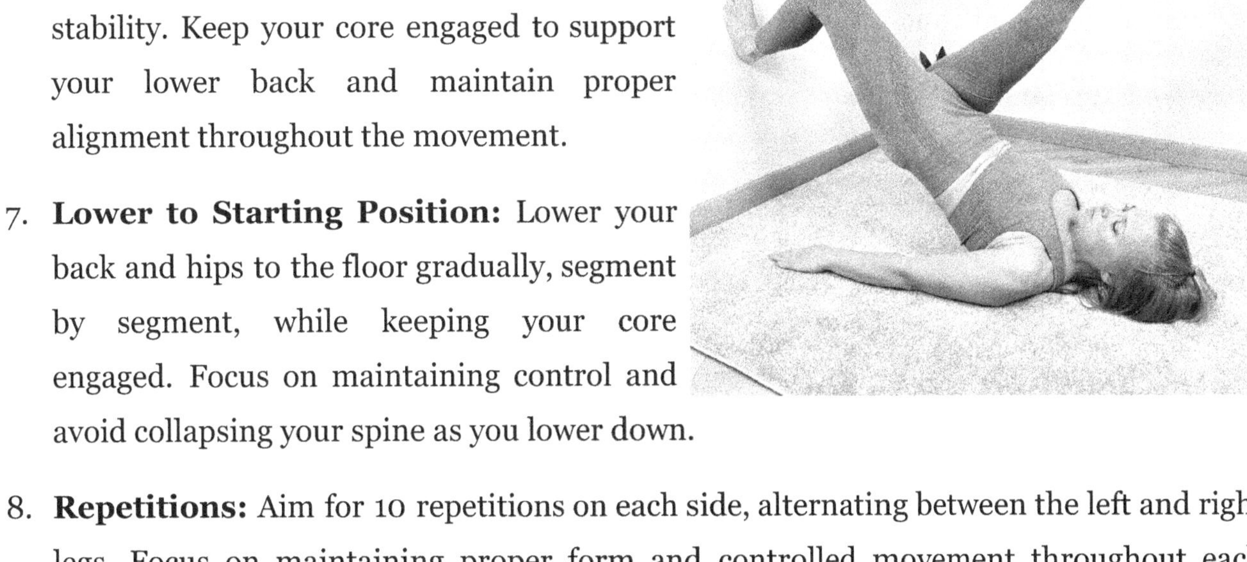

6. **Return to Midline:** Slowly bring your right leg back towards the midline of your body while maintaining control and pelvic stability. Keep your core engaged to support your lower back and maintain proper alignment throughout the movement.

7. **Lower to Starting Position:** Lower your back and hips to the floor gradually, segment by segment, while keeping your core engaged. Focus on maintaining control and avoid collapsing your spine as you lower down.

8. **Repetitions:** Aim for 10 repetitions on each side, alternating between the left and right legs. Focus on maintaining proper form and controlled movement throughout each repetition.

Warnings and Contraindications:

- Avoid overarching or rounding your lower back during the Single-Leg Bridge with Abduction exercise. Focus on maintaining a neutral spine alignment and engaging your core muscles to support your pelvis and lower back.
- Individuals with hip or knee injuries, pelvic instability, or any other medical conditions affecting the lower body should use caution when performing this exercise and may need to modify the range of motion or intensity to avoid exacerbating their condition.

Advanced Version:

- **Elevations with supporting foot:** Once you reach step number 5 of the exercise, add three lifts with the supporting foot against the wall, pushing with the toes and lifting the heel off the wall. Then, perform the alternate leg version.

8 Kneeling Side Leg Lift

Affected Area: Total body, with a focus on the core, hips, and outer thighs.

Objectives of the Exercise: The Kneeling Side Leg Lift exercise targets the muscles of the core, hips, and outer thighs, helping to improve stability, balance, and overall lower body strength. By isolating the lateral muscles of the hip and thigh, this exercise can help to enhance hip abduction strength and promote better alignment and function of the lower body.

Step-by-Step Instructions:

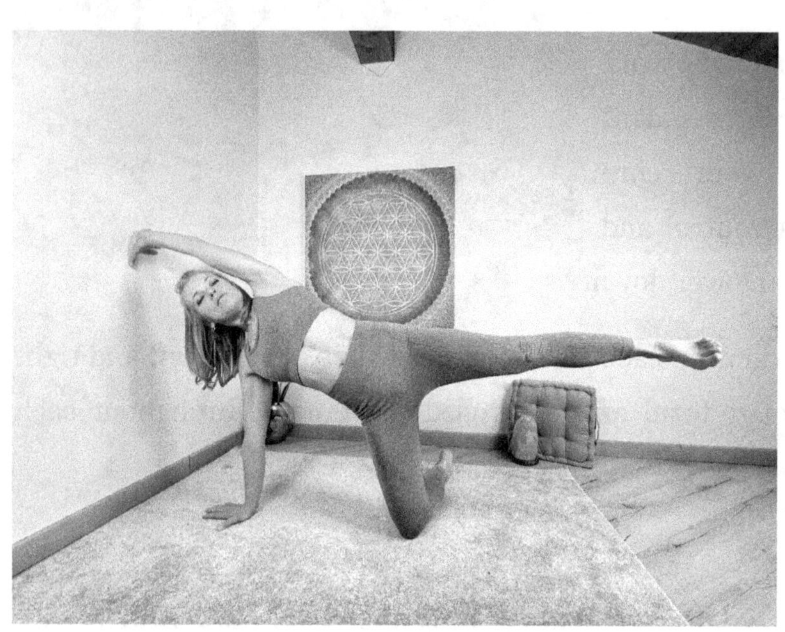

1. **Starting Position:** Begin by assuming a high-kneeling stance, orienting your left side toward the wall. Ensure your knees are directly beneath your hips, and your shins are vertical to the floor. Gradually lower your left side to the ground, positioning your left palm on the mat directly beneath your shoulder. Extend your right leg straight out to the side, planting your right foot firmly on the floor. For added comfort and stability, externally rotate your left knee by turning it slightly outward.

2. **Arm Position:** Raise your right arm over your head and place your right palm or fingertips on the wall. Do this while reaching your right arm up. Engage your triceps and obliques by gently pushing into the wall with your right arm. This action helps to stabilize your body and intensifies the engagement of the targeted muscles.

3. **Leg Lift:** Point your right toes and lift your right leg to approximately hip height, keeping it in line with your torso. Ensure that your hips remain stacked and your core stays engaged to maintain stability. Lower the right leg back down so that the toes hover just above the ground, maintaining control and smooth movement throughout.

4. **Breathing:** Breathe in as you lift your leg, and breathe out as you lower it back down. Focus on maintaining steady and controlled breathing throughout the exercise to enhance stability and concentration.

5. **Repetitions:** Perform 10 repetitions of the leg lift and lower on one side, focusing on proper form and controlled movement. Keep your core engaged and avoid any overarching or collapsing of the spine. After completing the set, switch sides and repeat the exercise sequence to ensure balanced muscle engagement and development.

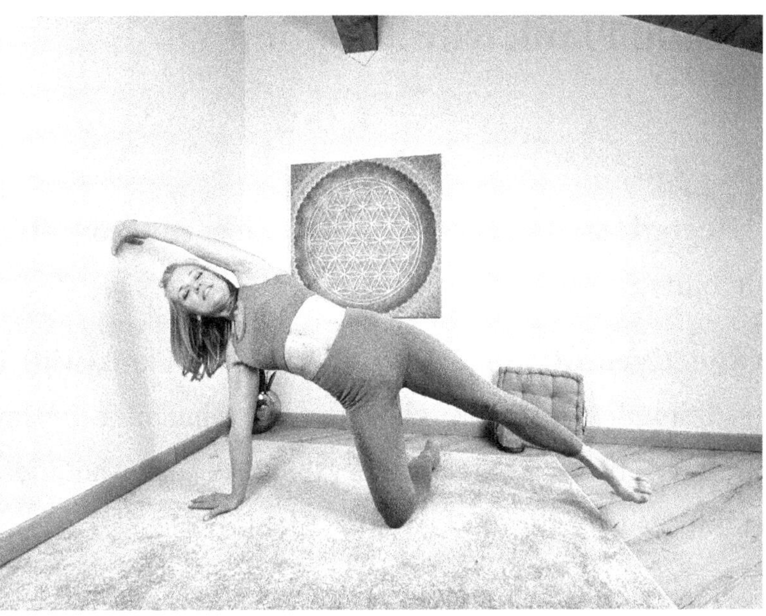

Warnings and Contraindications:

- Avoid overarching or collapsing of the spine during the Kneeling Side Leg Lift exercise. Remember to keep your spine in a neutral position and activate your core muscles to support your lower back and pelvis.
- Individuals with knee or hip injuries should use caution when performing this exercise and may need to modify the range of motion or intensity to avoid exacerbating their condition.

Advanced Version:

- **Extended Range of Motion:** Increase the range of motion by lifting your leg higher toward the ceiling while maintaining control and stability. Focus on engaging the core muscles to prevent overarching of the spine and ensure proper alignment. By challenging your muscles through a larger range of motion, you stimulate greater muscle fibers and enhance overall strength and flexibility.

9 Side Plank with Rotation

Affected Area: Total body, with a focus on core stability, shoulder strength, and rotational mobility.

Objectives of the Exercise: The Side Plank with Rotation is a dynamic variation of the traditional side plank, elevating the challenge by incorporating rotational movements. Its primary objectives are to strengthen the core, shoulders, and oblique muscles while improving stability, balance, and rotational mobility.

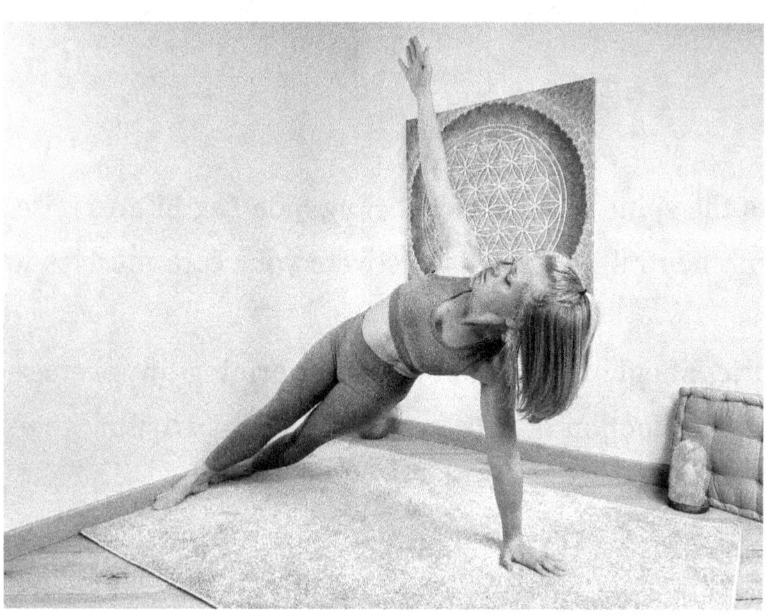

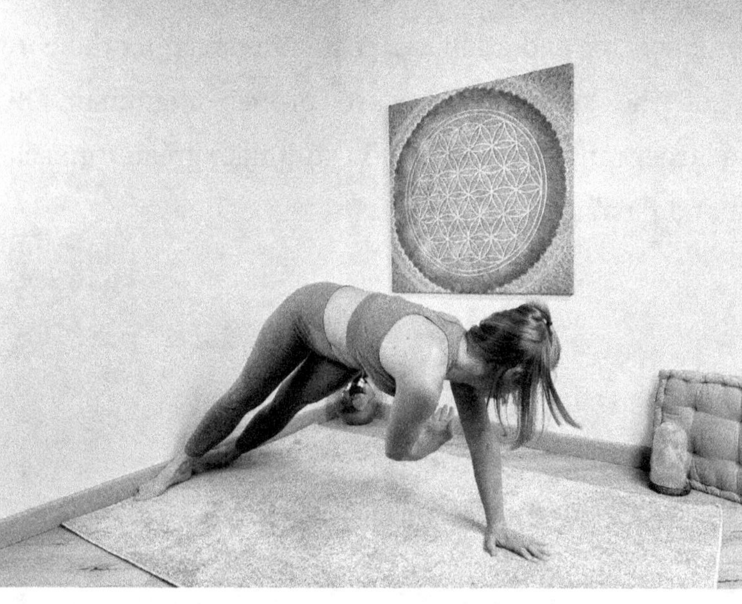

Step-by-Step Instructions:

1. **Starting Position:** Start by positioning yourself in front of the wall. Put your left palm firmly underneath your left shoulder, pressing it against the ground to support your body weight. Stagger your feet for stability, with your right foot positioned slightly ahead of your left foot, lean against the wall. Raise your hips from the ground, creating a straight line extending from your head to your heels.

2. **Extend the Arm:** Extend your right arm toward the ceiling, keeping it in line with your shoulder to initiate the side plank position. Ensure that your shoulder blades are engaged and your chest is open.

3. **Rotation Movement:** Slowly draw your right arm down and reach underneath your torso, looking to stretch it out as far as possible behind you.. Simultaneously, allow your torso to rotate,

pivoting on the support of your left arm and feet. Maintain elevated hips and an engaged core throughout the entire movement.

4. **Return to Side Plank:** Reverse the movement by opening back up into the side plank position, extending your right arm upward toward the ceiling. Focus on maintaining stability and control as you return to the starting position.

5. **Repeat:** Perform the rotation movement for a total of 10 repetitions, maintaining controlled movements and focusing on engaging your core throughout the exercise. Keep your breathing steady and rhythmic, inhaling as you rotate and exhaling as you return to the side plank position.

6. **Switch Sides:** Once you've completed the repetitions on one side, switch to the other side to ensure balanced muscle engagement and development. Repeat the exercise sequence with your right palm supporting your body weight and your left arm extended toward the ceiling.

Warnings and Contraindications:

- Avoid overarching or collapsing of the spine during the Side Plank with Rotation exercise. Concentrate on sustaining a straight line from your head to your heels, engaging your core muscles to provide support for your lower back.
- Individuals with shoulder injuries, wrist injuries, or any other medical conditions affecting the upper body should use caution when performing this exercise and may need to modify the range of motion or intensity to avoid exacerbating their condition.

Advanced Version:

- **Increase the repetitions:** to make the exercise more challenging, double the repetitions, so bring them up to 20 per side.

10 Reach Backs

Affected Area: Total body, with a focus on shoulders, arms, core, and flexibility.

Objectives of the Exercise: Reach Backs are designed to improve shoulder mobility, strengthen the arms and core, and enhance overall flexibility. This exercise targets multiple muscle groups simultaneously, providing a comprehensive workout for the entire body. The primary objectives include increasing range of motion in the shoulders, building upper body strength, and promoting better posture.

Step-by-Step Instructions:

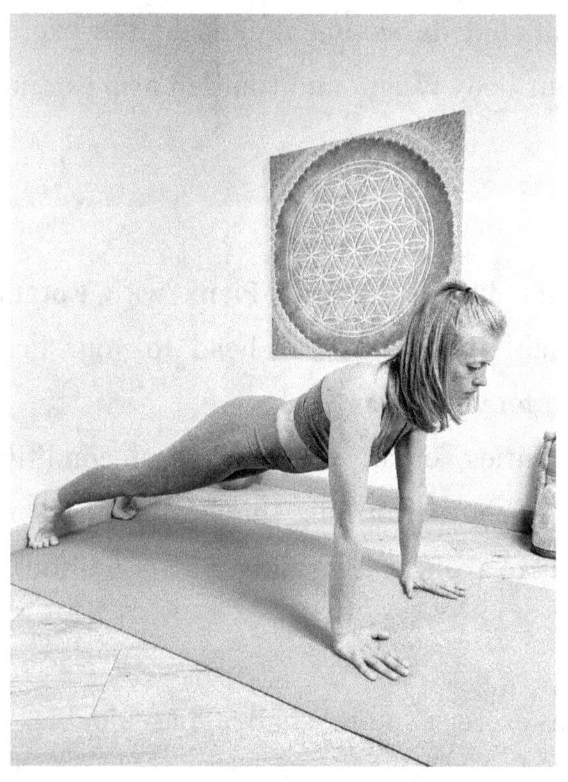
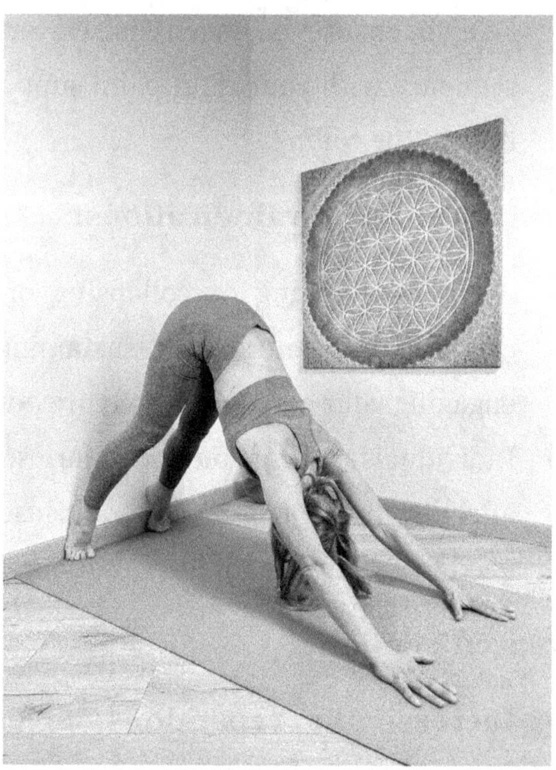

1. **Starting Position:** Commence in a high plank stance, placing your feet against the wall about as wide as a yoga mat. Confirm your wrists are directly beneath your shoulders, maintaining a straight line from your shoulders to your heels. Activate your core muscles to stabilize your body.

2. **Transition to Downward Dog:** Lift your hips upward and backward, transitioning into a Downward Dog position. Press your palms firmly into the ground and actively push your hips toward the ceiling. Allow your head to relax between your arms, and focus on elongating your spine. Take deep breaths to deepen the stretch.

3. **Reach Back with Right Hand:** Extend your right hand back, aiming to tap your left foot, ankle, or shin. Reach as far back as comfortably possible, feeling a stretch along the side of your body and through your shoulders and arms. Use the wall for support and stability as needed.

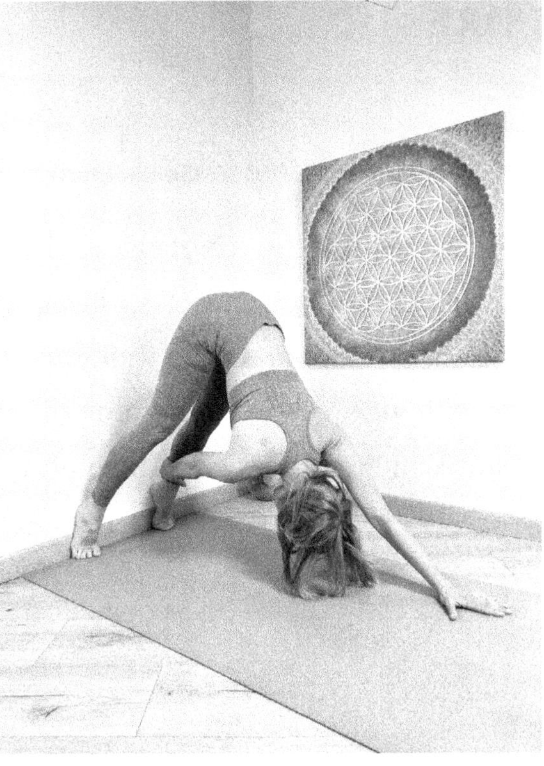

4. **Return to High Plank:** Shift your hips forward and downward, returning to the high plank position. Maintain a controlled descent, engaging your core muscles to prevent sagging in the lower back. Concentrate on sustaining correct form throughout the entirety of the exercise.

5. **Repeat on Opposite Side:** Extend your left hand back, aiming to tap your right foot, ankle, or shin. Reach as far back as you can while maintaining stability and control. Feel the stretch through the opposite side of your body and through your shoulders and arms.

6. **Perform Repetitions:** Alternate between reaching back with your right and left hands, performing 10 repetitions on each side. Focus on precision and control with each movement, emphasizing the stretch during each reach. Take your time and maintain a steady pace to maximize the advantages of the exercise.

Warnings and Contraindications:

- Ensure proper wrist alignment in the high plank position to prevent strain or injury to the wrists.
- Prevent overarching or rounding of your lower back throughout the movement. Concentrate on sustaining a neutral spine alignment and activate your core muscles for body stabilization.

Advanced Version:

- **Single-Leg Reach Back:** Lift one foot off the ground while reaching back with the opposite hand. This variation increases the challenge to your core muscles and balance, requiring greater stability and control throughout the movement.

Affected Area: Core muscles, such as the abdominals and lower back

Objectives of the Exercise: The Wall Plank primarily focuses on strengthening and stabilizing the core muscles, specifically targeting the abdominal region and lower back. Utilizing the support of the wall, this exercise offers a safe and effective method to engage the core without excessively straining the spine. Its main goal is to enhance core strength, improve posture, and enhance overall stability and balance.

Step-by-Step Instructions:

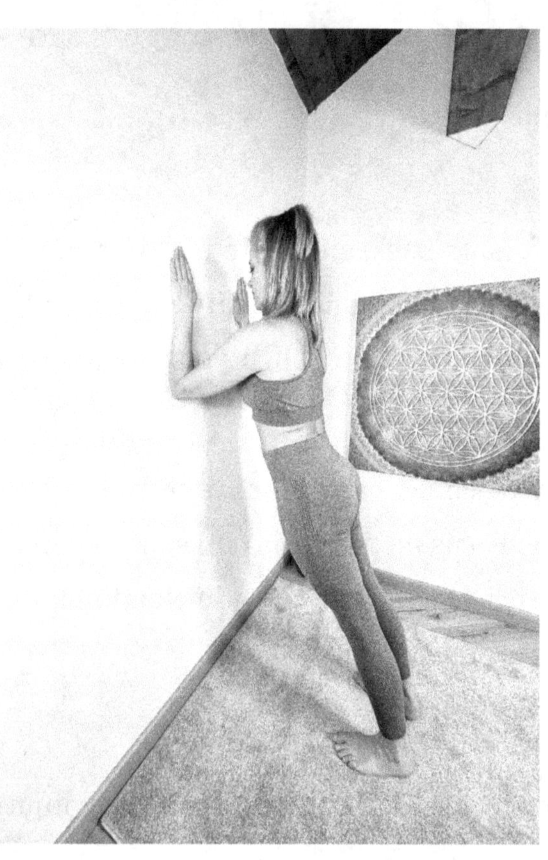

1. **Starting Position:** Commence standing facing the wall, maintaining a distance of approximately an arm's length. Position your hands on the wall at shoulder height, with a shoulder-width apart.

2. **Feet Position:** Step backward with your feet, ensuring they are hip-width apart. Your body should create a straight line from your head to your heels, resembling a plank position.

3. **Core Engagement:** Engage your core muscles by softly pulling your navel toward your spine, aiding in stabilizing your torso and activating the abdominal muscles.

4. **Body Alignment:** Ensure your body maintains a straight line, preventing excessive arching or sagging in the lower back. Concentrate on maintaining a neutral spine to prevent any strain or discomfort.

5. **Breathing and Focus:** While holding the plank position, concentrate on sustaining proper core engagement and controlled breathing. Initially, aim for a 20-30 second hold, progressively extending the duration as your strength and endurance improve with time.

Warnings and Contraindications:

- Individuals with existing shoulder, wrist, or back injuries should use caution when performing the Wall Plank exercise. Modify the position or seek guidance from a fitness professional if you experience any discomfort or pain during the exercise.
- Avoid holding your breath during the plank. Maintain a consistent breathing pattern to ensure adequate oxygenation to the muscles and prevent dizziness or lightheadedness.

Advanced Version:

- **Single-Leg Wall Plank:** Elevate one leg off the ground, maintaining a straight line from your head to your supporting foot. Hold this position for an extended duration, focusing on stability and balance. Alternate between legs to ensure balanced muscle engagement.

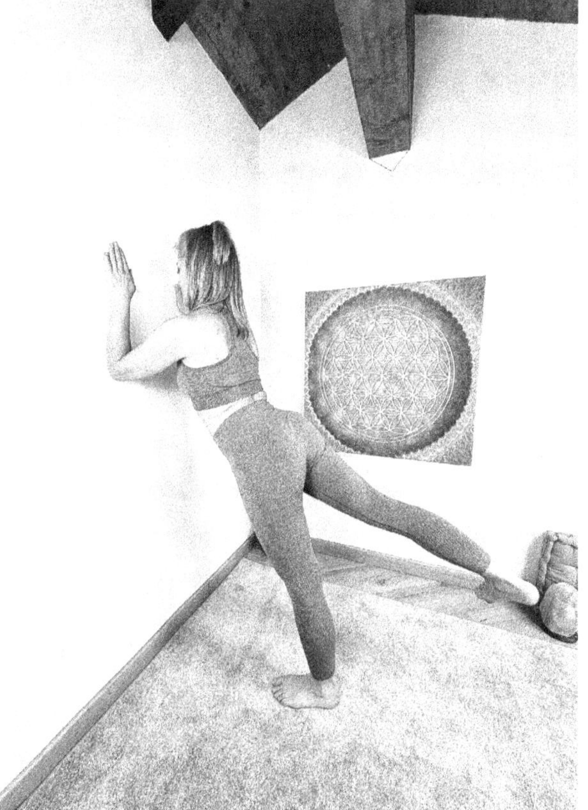

12 Wall Side Plank

Affected Area: Core muscles, particularly targeting the obliques and transverse abdominis.

Objectives of the Exercise: The Wall Side Plank is designed to strengthen and stabilize the core muscles, with a particular emphasis on the obliques and transverse abdominis. By utilizing the support of the wall, this exercise allows for focused engagement of the core while promoting proper form and alignment. The primary objectives include improving lateral stability, enhancing spinal alignment, and fortifying the muscles responsible for rotational movements.

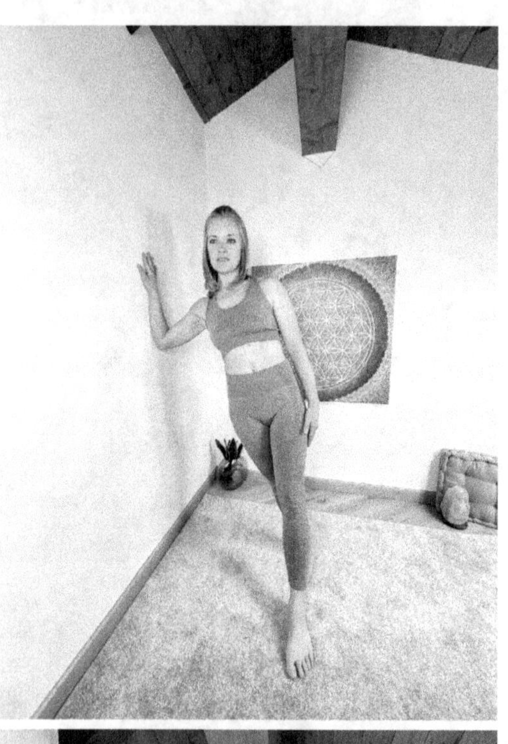

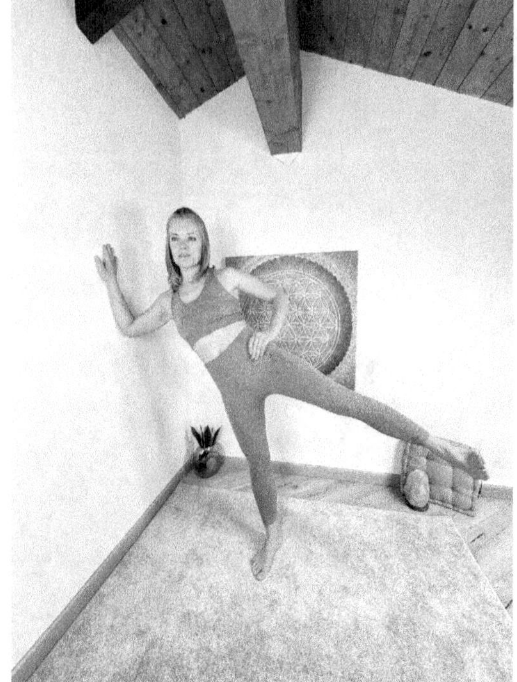

Step-by-Step Instructions:

1. **Starting Position:** Commence by standing sideways to the wall, ensuring that your right side faces the wall. Position your right forearm on the wall, perpendicular to your body.

2. **Leg Placement:** Extend your legs outwards, stacking your feet on top of each other or placing one foot in front of the other for added stability.

3. **Hip Lift:** Elevate your hips off the ground, ensuring that your body forms a straight line from your head to your heels. Maintain stability throughout the exercise by actively engaging your core muscles.

4. **Forearm Support:** Press your forearm into the wall for additional support, ensuring that your body remains aligned and your hips do not sag towards the ground.

5. **Hold and Breathe:** Maintain this position for 2/3 seconds, repeat for 10 times while maintaining a steady breathing rhythm.

6. **Repeat on Opposite Side:** Switch to the opposite side, ensuring equal engagement of both sides of the core.

Warnings and Contraindications:

- Individuals with wrist, elbow, or shoulder injuries should use caution when performing the Wall Side Plank. If you experience any discomfort or pain in these areas, discontinue the exercise and consult with a healthcare professional.
- Refrain from holding your breath during the exercise. Sustain a consistent breathing pattern by inhaling deeply through your nose and exhaling slowly through your mouth, promoting relaxation and focus.

Advanced Version:

- **Leg Lift Variation:** While holding the Wall Side Plank position, lift the top leg upward, maintaining proper alignment and stability. Hold the leg in the lifted position for 8 seconds before lowering it back down. Repeat the leg lift multiple times before switching sides. This variation adds an extra challenge by further engaging the muscles of the core and hips.

13 Wall Crunches

Affected Area: Core muscles, particularly targeting the rectus abdominis.

Objectives of the Exercise: Wall Crunches are aimed at fortifying the rectus abdominis and cultivating core strength, leading to enhanced abdominal stability. By elevating the head, shoulders, and upper back above the floor, this exercise effectively engages the core muscles, promoting comprehensive strength in the abdominal region.

Step-by-Step Instructions:

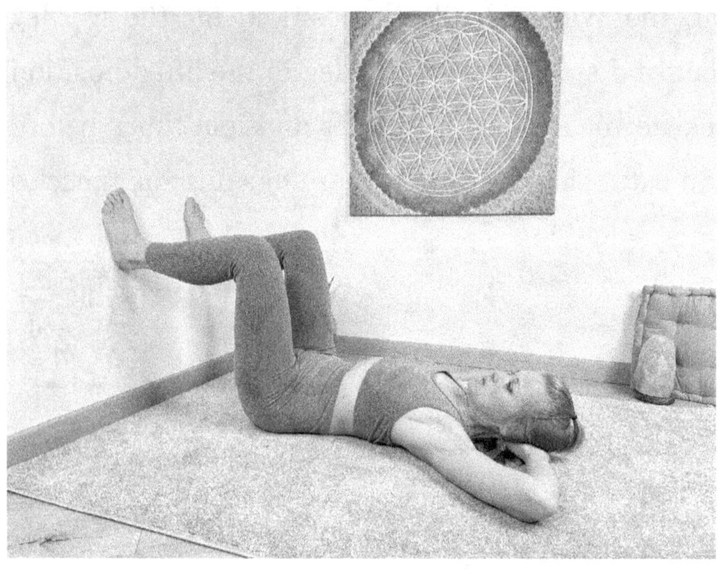

1. **Starting Position:** Begin by lying on your back with your feet against the wall. Bend your knees and position your feet flat on the wall. Your feet should be hip-width apart to provide a stable base of support. Support your neck gently with your fingertips behind your head, keeping your elbows wide to avoid straining the neck.

2. **Engage Core Muscles:** Activate the core muscles by drawing your navel towards your spine. This engagement will help stabilize your torso and create a solid foundation for the exercise.

3. **Initiate the Movement:** Elevate your head, shoulders, and upper back above the floor, initiating the movement by engaging your core muscles. Prioritize control throughout the entire range of motion, emphasizing the quality of each repetition over speed.

4. **Perform Crunches:** Execute traditional crunches by curling your upper body towards your knees. Concentrate on utilizing your core strength to raise your upper body while

ensuring your lower back remains firmly pressed against the floor. Refrain from pulling on your neck with your hands, as this action may lead to strain in the neck muscles.

5. **Range of Motion:** Lower your upper body back towards the floor, allowing your shoulder blades to lightly touch the ground before initiating the next repetition. Maintain a controlled movement pattern, emphasizing the contraction of the abdominal muscles with each crunch.

6. **Repetitions:** Perform 15-20 crunches to effectively engage the rectus abdominis and strengthen your core. Concentrate on upholding correct form and maintaining a steady breathing rhythm throughout the duration of the exercise.

Warnings and Contraindications:

- Avoid pulling on your neck with your hands during the crunches, as this can strain the neck muscles and lead to injury. Instead, focus on using your core strength to lift your upper body off the floor.
- If you have any pre-existing medical conditions or concerns related to abdominal strength or core stability, consult with a healthcare provider before attempting Wall Crunches or any other abdominal exercises.

Advanced Version:

- **Leg Raise Crunches:** Lift your legs off the wall and extend them towards the ceiling while performing the crunches. This variation increases the demand on the core muscles, especially the lower abdominals, and enhances overall stability and strength.

14 Wall 100s

Affected area: Core muscles

Objectives of the Exercise: The Wall 100s exercise is a dynamic core strengthening exercise that targets the abdominal muscles. It aims to improve core stability, endurance, and overall strength, while also enhancing coordination and control.

Step-by-Step Instructions:

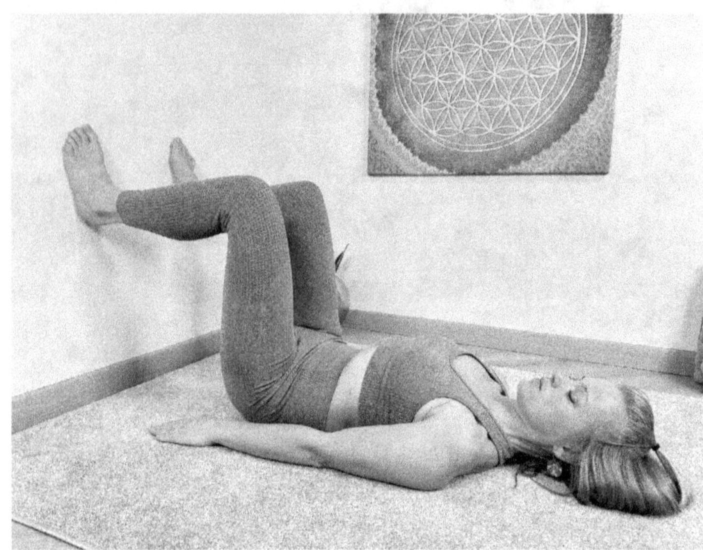

1. **Starting Position:** Commence by lying on your back with your knees bent and feet flat against a wall. Your knees and hips should be bent at approximately 90-degree angles, creating a rectangular shape beneath your knees. Ensure that your arms remain alongside your body with your palms facing downward.

2. **Engage Core:** Curl your head, shoulders, and upper back off the floor, engaging your abdominal muscles. Ensure your lower back remains pressed into the floor to maintain a neutral spine position.

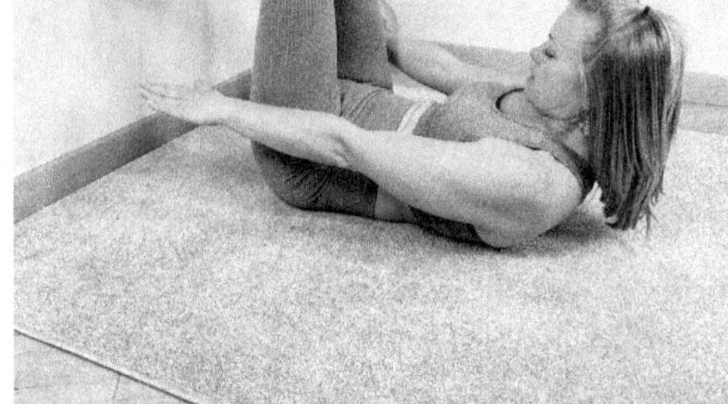

3. **Arm Position:** Extend your arms straight down by your sides, reaching toward your feet. Your fingertips should be pointing toward your feet, and your arms should remain in this position throughout the exercise.

4. **Breathing:** Take a deep inhalation through your nose to prepare for the motion.

5. **Movement:** Exhale slowly through your mouth as you begin making small, pulsing movements downward with your arms. Keep your arms straight

and tense as you press them down toward the floor, focusing on engaging your core muscles to stabilize your torso.

6. **Breathing Rhythm:** As you pulse your arms downward, take quick, short breaths, inhaling and exhaling rhythmically to maintain the pace of the movement.

7. **Finishing Position:** Continue pulsing your arms downward for a predetermined number of repetitions or for a set period, maintaining control and focus on engaging your core muscles throughout.

8. **Repetitions:** Perform the Wall 100s exercise for a predetermined number of repetitions, typically ranging from 10 to 100 pulses, depending on your fitness level and goals.

Warnings and Contraindications:

- Avoid straining your neck or shoulders during the Wall 100s exercise. Maintain relaxation in your neck and keep your shoulders away from your ears throughout the entire movement.
- Individuals with pre-existing neck or back conditions, such as herniated discs or spinal instability, should use caution when performing this exercise and may need to modify the range of motion or intensity to prevent exacerbating their condition.

Advanced Version:

- **Leg Variation:** Extend your legs straight up against the wall instead of keeping them bent. This increases the lever arm and requires greater core strength and stability to maintain the position while performing the arm pulses.

15 Toe Touches

Affected Area: Core muscles (abdominals, obliques).

Objectives of the Exercise: Toe Touches are aimed at strengthening the core muscles, especially the abdominals and obliques, while also improving flexibility in the hamstrings. This exercise helps to enhance overall core stability, posture, and spinal alignment.

Step-by-Step Instructions:

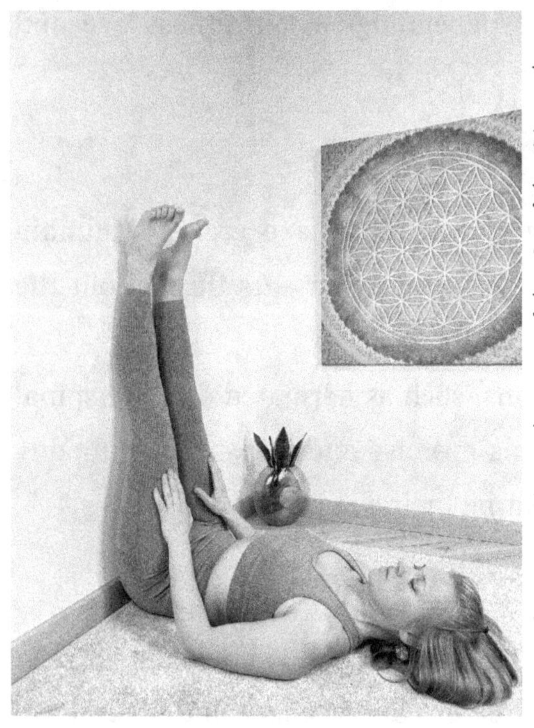

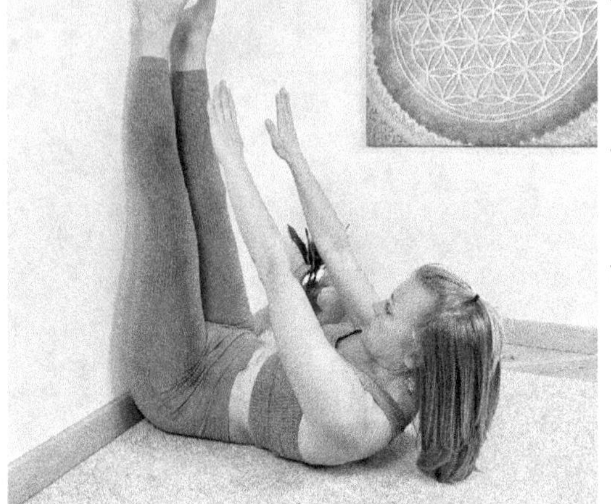

1. **Starting Position:** Lie on your back with your buttocks near the wall and your legs extended upward, resting against the wall. Keep your arms comfortably by your sides with palms facing down. Engage the abdominal muscles by gently drawing your navel toward your spine and pressing your lower back into the floor.

2. **Leg Position:** Extend your legs upward against the wall, ensuring they are straight and close together. Flex your feet so that your toes point toward the ceiling.

3. **Breathing:** Breathe in deeply through your nose, expanding your ribcage and filling your lungs with air.

4. **Movement:** Exhale slowly through your mouth as you activate your core muscles to lift your head, neck, and shoulders off the floor. Simultaneously, reach your hands toward your toes, aiming to touch them or come as close as possible while maintaining control and without straining.

5. **Reaching Up:** Continue reaching toward your toes until you feel a gentle stretch in your hamstrings and a contraction in your abdominal muscles. Focus on keeping your lower back pressed into the floor to avoid overarching.

6. **Hold and Lower:** Hold the lifted position for a moment, feeling the engagement in your core muscles.

Then, inhale as you slowly lower your head, neck, and shoulders back down to the floor, returning to the starting position with control.

7. **Repetitions:** Aim to complete 10-12 repetitions of Toe Touches, focusing on quality over quantity and maintaining proper form throughout each repetition.

Warnings and Contraindications:

- Avoid straining your neck or shoulders during the Toe Touches exercise. Focus on using your abdominal muscles to lift your head, neck, and shoulders off the floor, rather than pulling with your arms.
- Individuals with pre-existing back or neck conditions, such as herniated discs or spinal instability, should use caution when performing this exercise and may need to modify the range of motion or intensity to avoid exacerbating their condition.

Advanced Version:

- **While lifted perform pulses**: In the raised position, perform 4 or more pulses to increase muscle tension, repeat for 10 times.

16 Wall Bicycle

Affected Area: Core muscles, particularly targeting the rectus abdominis and obliques.

Objectives of the Exercise: The Wall Bicycle exercise is a dynamic variation of the traditional bicycle crunch, tailored to target and strengthen the core muscles with the added support of a wall. This variation offers an excellent entry point for beginners, providing stability and assistance during the movement. The primary focus is on engaging the rectus abdominis and obliques, contributing to improved core strength and stability. Additionally, the exercise involves the hip flexors, making it a comprehensive workout for the abdominal region.

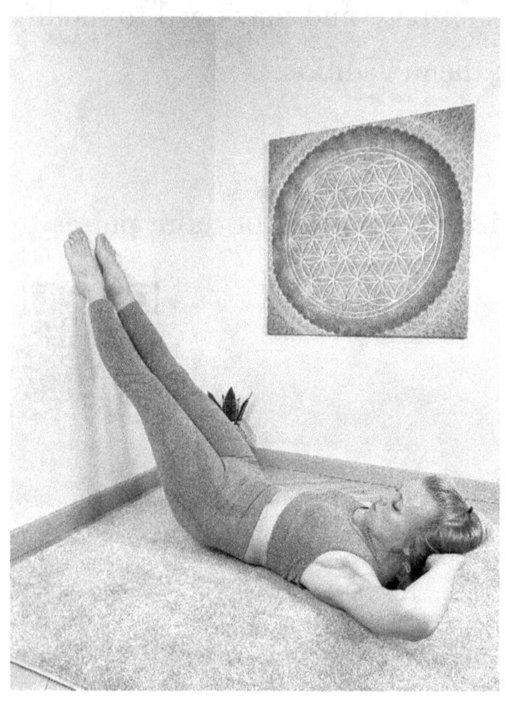

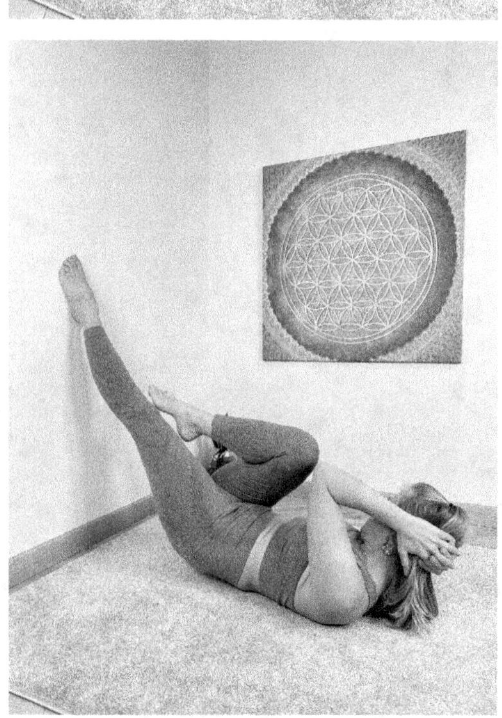

Step-by-Step Instructions:

1. **Starting Position:** Commence by lying on your back on a comfortable surface, positioning your buttocks close to a wall. Extend your legs upward, pressing your feet against the wall with your knees slightly bent. This position ensures stability and support during the exercise.

2. **Hand Placement:** Put your hands lightly behind your head, interlocking your fingers. Keep your elbows pointed outward and relaxed to avoid straining the neck and shoulders.

3. **Engage Core Muscles:** Tighten your abdominal muscles by drawing your navel toward your spine. This engagement helps stabilize your core and prepares it for the upcoming movement.

4. **Lift Head and Shoulders:** Gently lift your head and shoulders off the floor, ensuring that your lower back maintains contact with the mat. This initial lift establishes the starting position for the exercise.

5. **Pedaling Motion:** Lift your right leg off the wall, bringing your knee toward your chest. At the same time, rotate your upper body to the right, bringing your left elbow closer to your right knee. This motion resembles the pedaling action of riding a bicycle.

6. **Leg Extension:** As you rotate and bring your knee and elbow together, extend your left leg straight out, keeping it elevated above the floor. This extension engages the muscles of the core and legs, increasing the intensity of the exercise.

7. **Alternate Sides:** Reverse the movement by bringing your right elbow closer to your left knee, simultaneously extending your right leg straight out. Continue to alternate sides, performing the bicycle motion with your legs while keeping your feet on the wall.

8. **Repetitions:** Aim for 12-15 repetitions on each side, or adjust based on your comfort and fitness level. Perform the exercise at a steady pace, focusing on controlled movements and maintaining proper form throughout the entire sequence.

Warnings and Contraindications:

- Avoid tugging on your neck with your hands while performing the exercise, as this may strain the neck muscles and lead to injury. Focus instead on activating your abdominal muscles to lift your head and shoulders off the floor.
- If you have any pre-existing medical conditions or concerns related to abdominal strength or core stability, consult with a healthcare provider before attempting the Wall Bicycle exercise or any other abdominal exercises.

Advanced Version:

- **Variation With Abdominal:** After each pedal stroke, when your legs are extended and resting, both against the wall, arch your back trying to bring yourself closer to your pelvis while performing an abdominal exercise.

17 Lying Windshield Wipers

Affected Area: Core muscles, including the abdomen, obliques, and lower back.

Objectives of the Exercise: Lying Windshield Wipers is an effective core exercise that targets the muscles of the abdomen, obliques, and lower back. By incorporating controlled leg movements while lying on your back with the support of the wall, this exercise increases core strength, stability, and flexibility. The name "Windshield Wipers" aptly describes the lateral leg movement, resembling the motion of windshield wipers in a car.

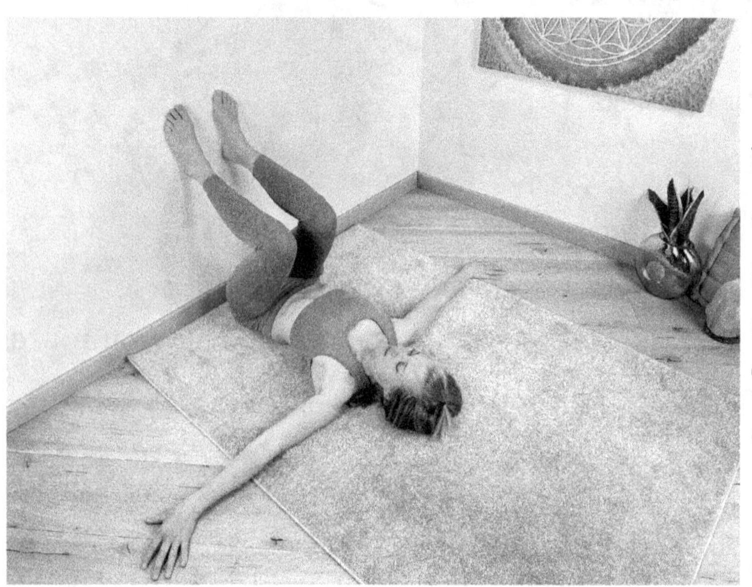

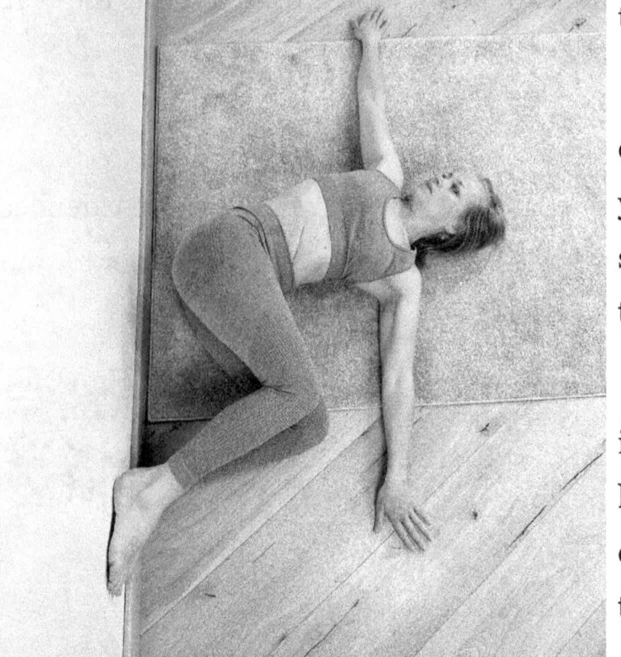

Step-by-Step Instructions:

1. **Starting Position:** Lie on your back with your rear close to the wall, ensuring that your knees are bent at a 90-deg. angle and your feet are flat against the wall, touching each other. This position provides stability and engages the core from the beginning.

2. **Arm Positioning:** Extend your arms out to your sides, creating a T-shape with your body. This arm positioning enhances balance and stability during the leg movements, allowing you to maintain control throughout the exercise.

3. **Engage Core Muscles:** Breathe in deeply and engage your core muscles by drawing your navel toward your spine. This engagement stabilizes your torso and prepares your core for the upcoming movement.

4. **Lower Legs to the Left:** On your next inhale, slowly lower both your legs down to your left side until your knees touch the floor. Sustain contact between your feet and the wall throughout the movement to guarantee stability and maintain proper alignment.

5. **Return to Center:** Exhale as you use your core muscles to bring your torso back to the center position. Focus on twisting your hips and engaging your obliques to control the movement. Refrain from using momentum or swinging your legs to maintain stability and maximize the effectiveness of the exercise.

6. **Lower Legs to the Right:** Breathe in again, lowering both your legs down to your right side until your knees touch the floor. Keep your movements controlled and deliberate, focusing on engaging the core muscles rather than the lower back.

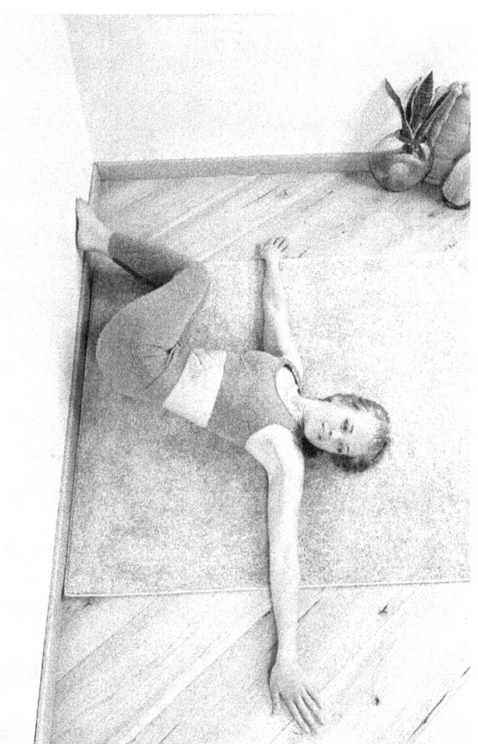

7. **Return to Center:** Exhale and use your core muscles to bring your torso back to the center position. To optimize the benefits for your core muscles, ensure you maintain proper form and alignment throughout the entire movement.

8. **Repeat:** Continue alternating between lowering your legs to the left and right sides, performing the twisting motion with each repetition. Aim for a total of 20 full repetitions, or adjust based on your comfort and fitness level.

Warnings and Contraindications:

- Avoid over-twisting the torso or allowing the lower back to arch excessively during the movement. Focus on engaging the core muscles to control the motion and maintain proper alignment throughout the exercise.

- If you have any pre-existing medical conditions or concerns related to core strength or flexibility, consult with a healthcare provider before attempting Lying Windshield Wipers or any other core exercises.

Advanced Version:

- **Extended Leg Variation:** Instead of keeping your knees bent at a 90-degree angle, straighten your legs upward toward the ceiling. This variation increases the lever length, intensifying the engagement of the core muscles and challenging your stability and control.

18 Wall Twist

Affected Area: Core muscles, particularly targeting the obliques and deep core muscles.

Objectives of the Exercise: Wall Twist is a dynamic Pilates exercise that ignites core strength with precision. This movement combines the challenge of rotational twists with the support of the wall, creating an effective workout for the abdominal muscles. By lifting your legs slightly off the floor and maintaining contact with the wall, Wall Twist intensifies the engagement of your core, promoting both strength and flexibility. This exercise targets the obliques and deep core muscles, contributing to a sculpted midsection and improved rotational mobility.

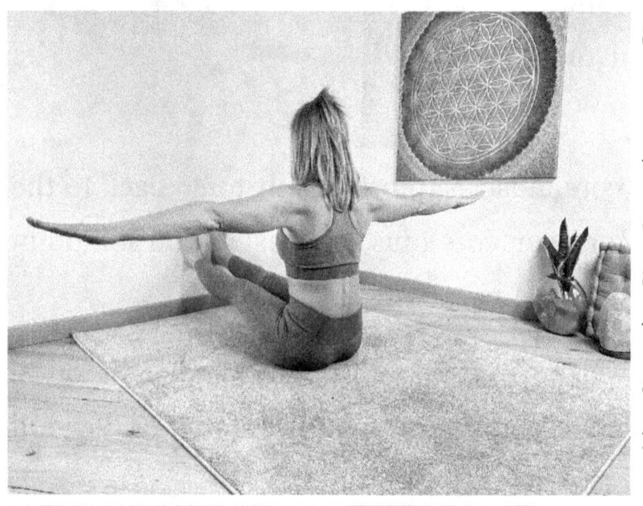

Step-by-Step Instructions:

1. **Starting Position:** Sit in front of a wall with your legs extended straight in front of you and slightly lifted off the floor. Ensure that the soles of your feet are pressed against the wall, with your legs spread wide apart. Extend your arms out to the sides at shoulder height, maintaining a straight and upright posture.

2. **Engage Core Muscles:** Activate your core muscles by drawing your navel toward your spine. This engagement stabilizes your torso and prepares your core for the rotational movement.

3. **Initiate Rotation:** From the starting position, begin a controlled rotation towards one side of your body. Keep your legs lifted off the floor and maintain contact between the soles of your feet and the wall. Focus on using your obliques to initiate the twist while keeping your upper body tall and your spine straight.

4. **Hold and Contract:** Once you reach the end of the rotation, hold the position for approximately 1 second, emphasizing the contraction of your oblique muscles. Ensure that your legs remain lifted and your feet stay in contact with the wall throughout the movement.

5. **Return to Center:** Slowly and deliberately return to the starting position, maintaining control over the movement. Keep your core engaged and your spine aligned as you rotate back to the center.

6. **Alternate Sides:** Repeat the rotation, this time towards the opposite side of your body. Hold the rotated position for 1 second before returning to the center. Alternate between rotations to each side, focusing on maintaining proper form and control throughout the exercise.

7. **Repetitions:** Perform the Wall Twist for the specified number of repetitions, typically aiming for 10-15 rotations to each side. Prioritize precision and control over the number of repetitions, focusing on executing each movement with quality.

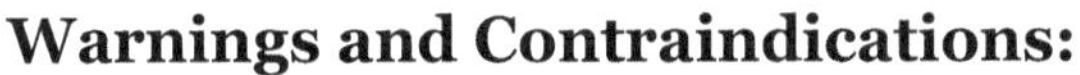

Warnings and Contraindications:

- Avoid over-twisting the torso or allowing the lower back to arch excessively during the movement. Focus on engaging the core muscles to control the rotation and maintain proper spinal alignment throughout the exercise.
- If you have any pre-existing medical conditions or concerns related to core strength or spinal mobility, consult with a healthcare provider before attempting Wall Twist or any other rotational core exercises.

Advanced Version:

- **Single-Leg Variation:** Lift one leg off the wall and hold it in the air while performing the rotations. This variation increases the instability and requires greater activation of the core muscles to maintain balance and control throughout the exercise.

19 Marching Bridge

Affected Area: Core muscles, glutes, hip flexors, and lower body.

Objectives of the Exercise: The Marching Bridge is designed to strengthen the core muscles while also targeting the glutes, hip flexors, and lower body. This exercise aims to enhance stability, improve balance, and promote proper alignment, contributing to overall body strength and flexibility.

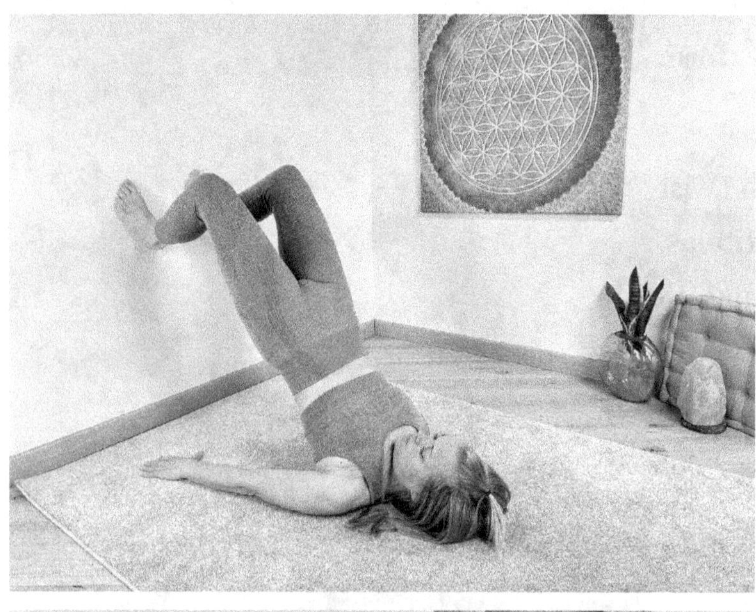

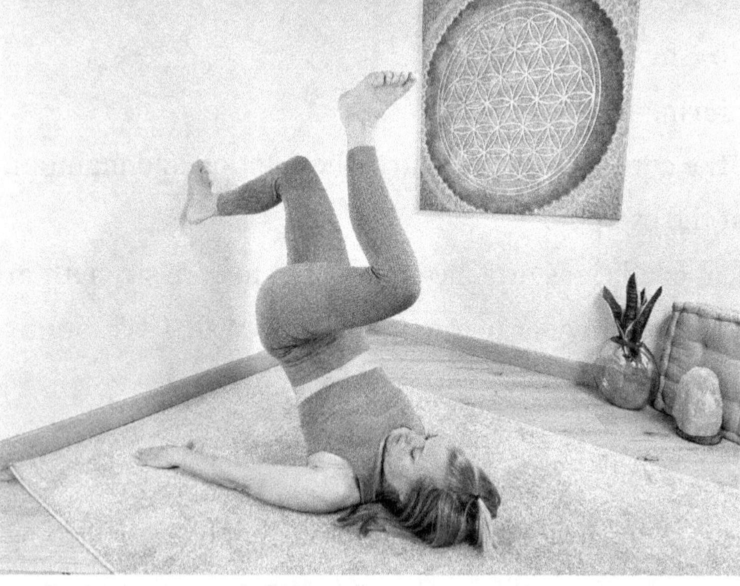

Step-by-Step Instructions:

1. **Starting Position:** Sit approximately one foot away from the wall, lying down on your back. Put your feet flat against the wall, creating a tabletop position with your legs bent at a 90-degree angle. Ensure that your arms rest comfortably at your sides.

2. **Hip Lift:** Press firmly through your feet against the wall to lift your hips off the floor. Ensure that your body forms a straight line from your shoulders to your knees. Maintain a neutral spine, avoiding any arching in your lower back. This position marks the starting point for the exercise.

3. **Marching Motion:** With an emphasis on stability, lift your left foot off the floor, bringing your knee toward your chest. Maintain the bend in your knee, solely moving at the hip joint until your thigh is perpendicular to your torso. This controlled marching motion isolates the left leg.

4. **Reverse and Repeat:** Reverse the motion, gently lowering your left foot back to the wall, completing one repetition. Ensure a smooth and deliberate movement, focusing on engagement in your core and stability in your hips.

5. **Alternate Legs:** Repeat the same marching motion with your right leg, lifting the knee toward your chest and then lowering it back to the wall. Continue alternating between left and right legs to perform a set of repetitions.

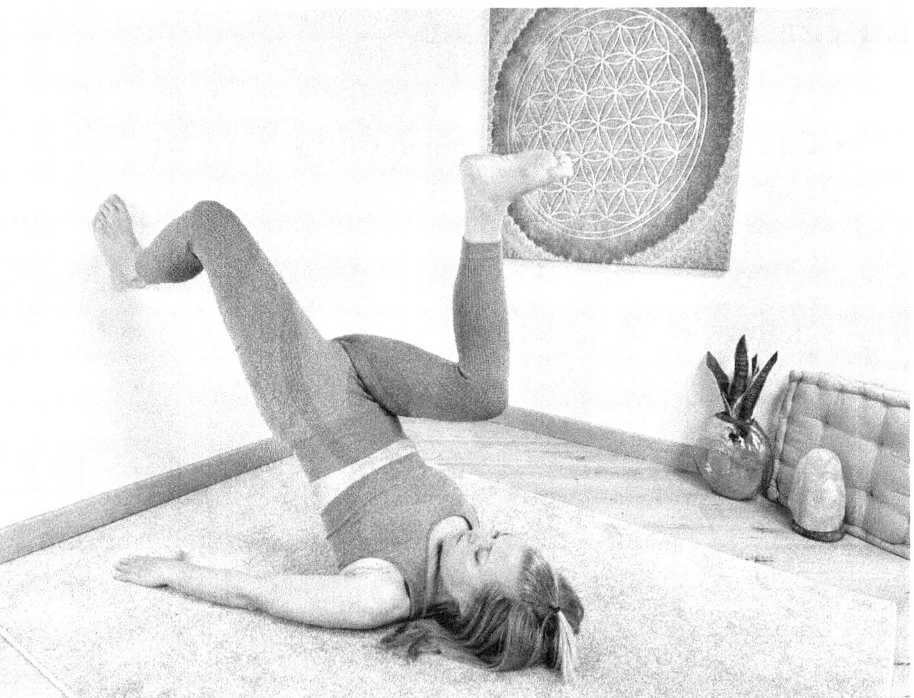

6. **Repetitions:** Aim to perform 10 repetitions with each leg, maintaining a consistent pace and emphasizing precision in each movement. The controlled nature of the Marching Bridge enhances its effectiveness in targeting specific muscle groups.

Warnings and Contraindications:

- Avoid overarching your lower back during the lifting phase of the exercise. Focus on engaging your core muscles to maintain proper spinal alignment and stability throughout the movement.
- If you have any concerns or medical conditions related to core strength, hip mobility, or lower body stability, consult with a healthcare provider before attempting the Marching Bridge or any other similar exercises.

Advanced Version:

- **Leg extension variation:** Instead of keeping the knee bent at a 90-degree angle when bringing the thigh towards the torso, fully extend the leg and try to bring the foot as close to the floor as possible.

20 Standing Knee Raises

Affected Area: Core, legs, and hip flexors.

Objectives of the Exercise: Standing Knee Raises are designed to strengthen the core muscles, especially the abdominals, while also engaging the legs and hip flexors. This exercise helps improve balance, stability, and coordination. The primary objectives include building core strength, enhancing balance, and developing better control over leg movements.

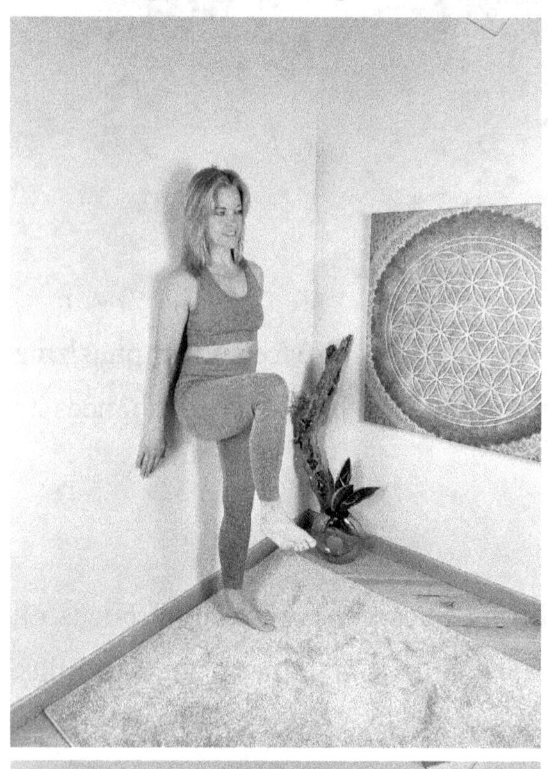

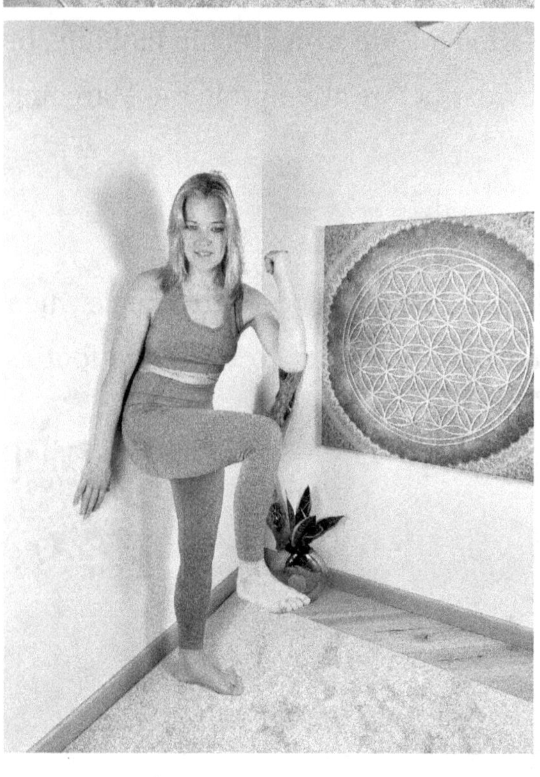

Step-by-Step Instructions:

1. **Starting Position:** Stand with your back against the wall, ensuring good posture with shoulders relaxed and chest lifted. Put your hands on your hips to stabilize your upper body.

2. **Feet Position:** Open your legs to about shoulder-width apart. This stance provides a stable base for the exercise and ensures balance throughout the movement.

3. **Lift Right Leg:** Breathe in deeply, and as you breathe out, lift your right leg off the floor, bending your knee to a 90-degree angle. Keep your foot flexed, with toes pointing toward the ceiling.

4. **Crunch Movement:** At the same time as you lift your right leg, slightly bend your left shoulder toward your elevated right knee. This creates a slight crunching motion in your abdominal muscles, engaging the core.

5. **Hold and Contract:** Hold the raised position for a brief moment, focusing on the contraction in your core and hip flexors. This pause enhances the effectiveness of the exercise.

6. **Return to Starting Position:** Lower your right leg back to the floor in a controlled manner,

keeping the movement smooth and deliberate. Return to the starting position with both feet on the ground and hands on your hips.

7. **Repeat with Left Leg:** Repeat the same movement with your left leg. Breathe in as you lift your left leg, bending the knee to a 90-degree angle. Simultaneously, bend your right shoulder toward your elevated left knee, engaging the abdominal muscles.

8. **Alternate Legs:** Continue alternating between lifting your right and left legs while performing the slight crunching motion with the opposite shoulder. Each lift and crunch counts as one repetition.

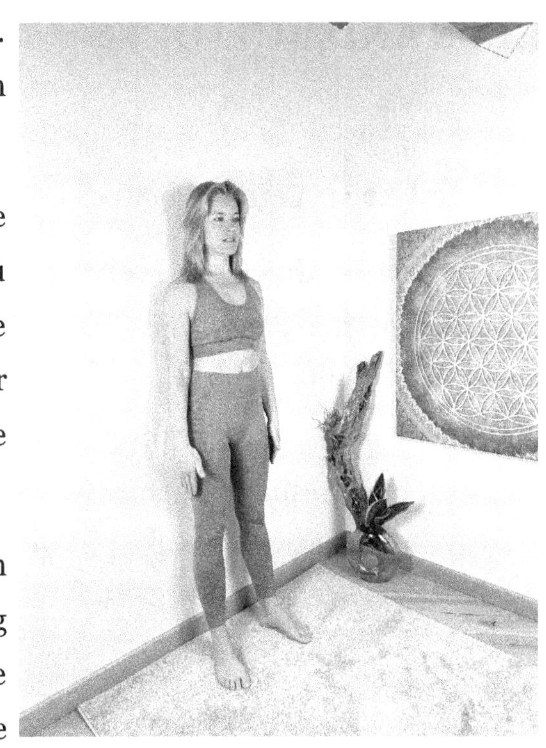

9. **Complete Repetitions:** Aim to complete 20 repetitions in total, alternating between each leg. This means 10 repetitions per leg. Maintain a steady pace, focusing on controlled movements and proper form throughout the exercise.

Warnings and Contraindications:

- Ensure proper form throughout the exercise to avoid straining the lower back or hip joints.
- Avoid jerky or rapid movements, as this can lead to loss of balance or strain on the muscles.

Advanced Version:

- **High Knee Hold:** Instead of returning the leg to the floor after each raise, hold the knee in the raised position for a few seconds before lowering it down. This increases the time under tension for the core muscles, enhancing their endurance and strength.

Affected Area: Legs and buttocks.

Objectives of the Exercise: Wall Squats target and tone the muscles of the lower body, focusing on the quadriceps, hamstrings, and glutes. This exercise enhances lower body strength, stability, and endurance, thereby improving athletic performance and functional movement patterns. By incorporating Wall Squats into your workout routine, you can build stronger, more resilient leg muscles while also promoting proper alignment and posture.

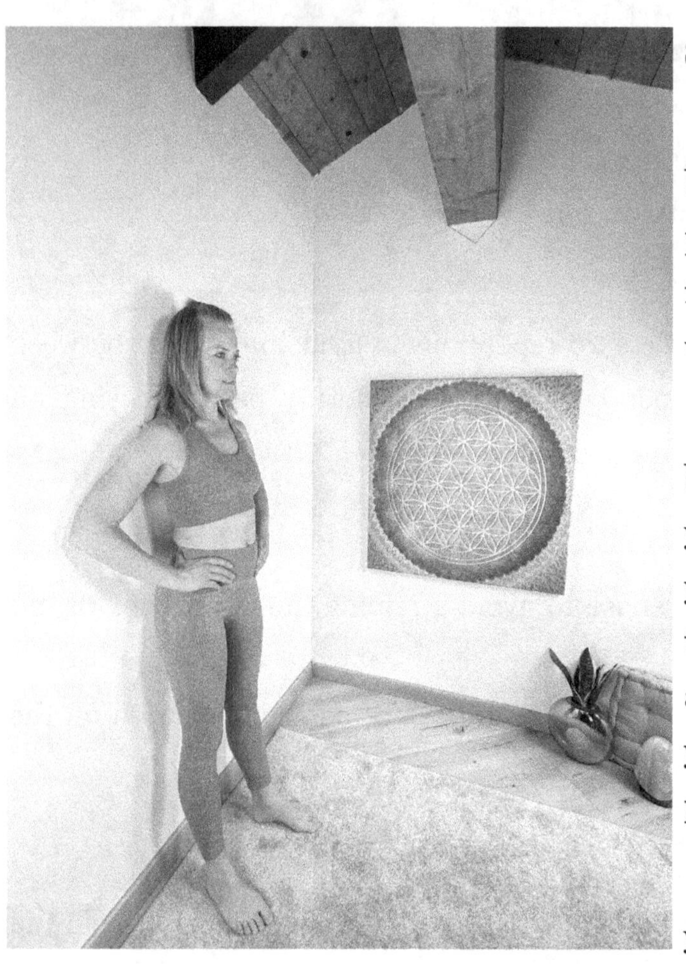

Step-by-Step Instructions:

1. **Starting Position:** Stand with your back against a sturdy wall and your feet positioned hip-width apart. Ensure that your feet are a comfortable distance away from the wall to allow for proper movement.17

2. **Lowering Phase:** Slowly lower your body down the wall, bending your knees as if you're sitting into an invisible chair. Keep your back firmly against the wall throughout the movement to maintain proper spinal alignment. Your knees should be in line with your ankles, and your thighs should be parallel to the ground.

3. **Breathing:** Breathe in as you lower yourself down into the squat position. Focus on deep, diaphragmatic breathing to oxygenate your muscles and support your movements.

4. **Hold Position:** Hold the squat position for a few seconds, focusing on engaging the muscles of your legs and buttocks. Keep your core muscles engaged to uphold stability and balance.

5. **Breathing:** Exhale as you push through your heels and return to the starting position. Keep the movement controlled and deliberate, emphasizing the engagement of your leg muscles.

6. **Repetitions:** Aim to complete 12 to 15 repetitions of the Wall Squat. Focus on maintaining proper form and alignment throughout each repetition. As you become more comfortable with the exercise, you can gradually increase the number of repetitions or add resistance to further challenge your muscles.

Warnings and Contraindications:

- Avoid rounding your lower back or allowing your knees to extend beyond your toes during the Wall Squat. These movements can place excessive strain on the joints and increase the risk of injury.
- Individuals with balance issues or difficulty standing for prolonged periods should exercise caution when performing Wall Squats. Use a support such as a chair or stability ball if needed to maintain balance and stability during the exercise.

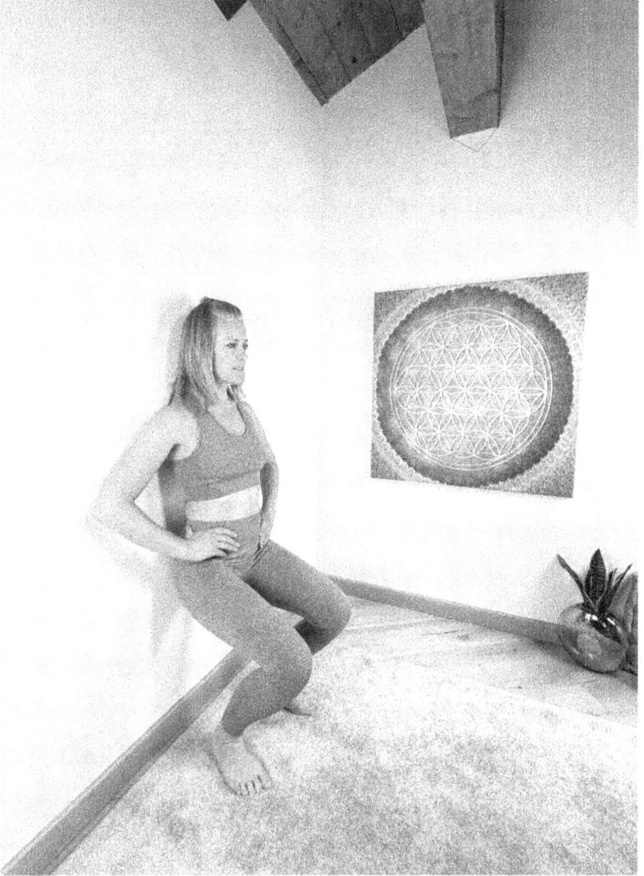

Advanced Version:

- **Extend the holding time:** to further advance and strengthen the targeted areas, once you've reached the squat position, hold it for 10 seconds. This will take the exercise to the next level.

22 Split Squats

Affected Area: Legs (quadriceps, hamstrings) and buttocks (glutes).

Objectives of the Exercise: Split Squats are a dynamic lower body exercise aimed at targeting the muscles of the legs and buttocks. This exercise helps to improve lower body strength, stability, and balance while also enhancing flexibility in the hip flexors and improving overall lower body function.

Step-by-Step Instructions:

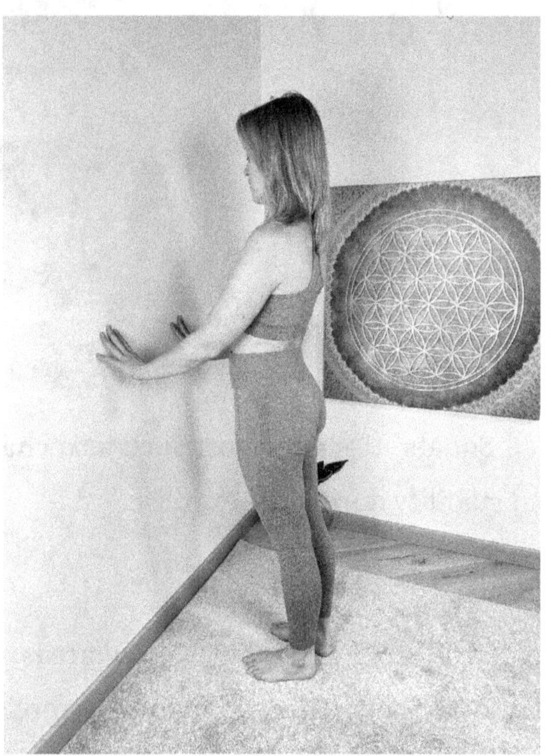
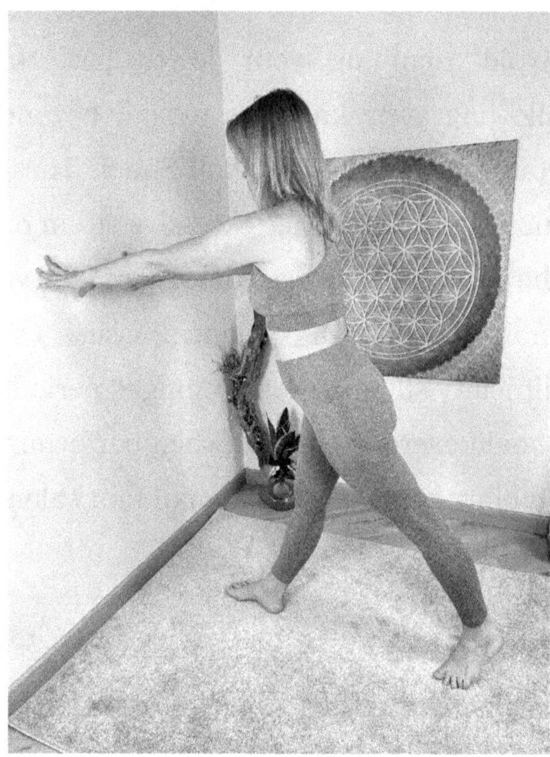

1. **Starting Position:** You are standing in front of the wall. Place your hands on the wall to use it as support. Your feet are side by side.

2. **Breathing:** Breathe deeply through your nose, expanding your chest as you fill your lungs with air.

3. **Movement:** Slowly exhale through the mouth as you step back with your left leg, lowering your body towards the ground by bending both knees. Lower yourself towards the floor, ensuring that the front knee does not extend beyond the toes and keeping the back knee facing downwards.

4. **Squatting Down:** Continue lowering your body until your front thigh is parallel to the floor, or as close to parallel as possible, while maintaining a straight back and upright

torso. Concentrate on maintaining engagement in your core muscles and keeping your chest lifted throughout the entire movement.

5. **Hold and Push Up:** Hold the lowered position for a moment, feeling the engagement in your front leg muscles. Then, breathe out as you push through your front heel to return to the starting position, straightening your front leg and bringing your back leg forward to meet it.

6. **Repetitions:** Complete 10-12 repetitions of Split Squats on one side before switching to the other side. Alternate between legs for each set, maintaining proper form and control throughout each repetition.

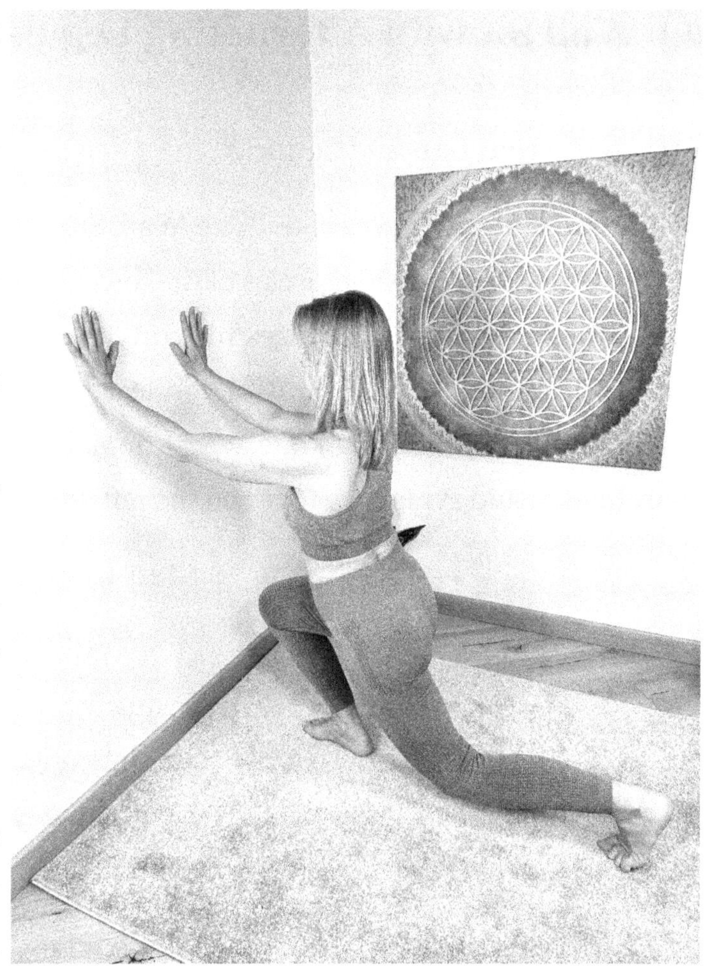

Warnings and Contraindications:

- Avoid allowing your front knee to collapse inward or extend past your toes during the Split Squats. Keep your knee aligned with your ankle to prevent strain or injury.
- Individuals with knee or hip issues, such as arthritis or ligament injuries, should use caution when performing this exercise and may need to modify the range of motion or intensity to avoid exacerbating their condition.

Advanced Version:

- **Increase the duration of the flexion:** Perform the exercise by increasing the flexion time, bringing it to at least 10 seconds. This way, it strengthens the leg muscles, thighs, and back more effectively.

23 Wall Sit with Alternating Leg Extension

Affected Area: Legs and buttocks.

Objectives of the Exercise: The Wall Sit with Alternating Leg Extension is designed to target and strengthen the muscles of the lower body, especially the quadriceps, hamstrings, and glutes. This exercise also engages the core muscles for stability and balance. By combining the static hold of a wall sit with dynamic leg extensions, it helps improve lower body strength, endurance, and muscle tone. Additionally, the alternating leg movement enhances coordination and symmetry between the left and right sides of the body.

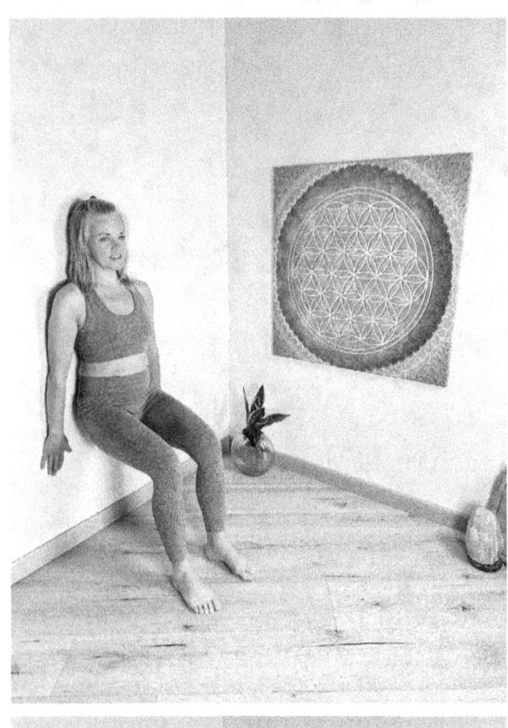

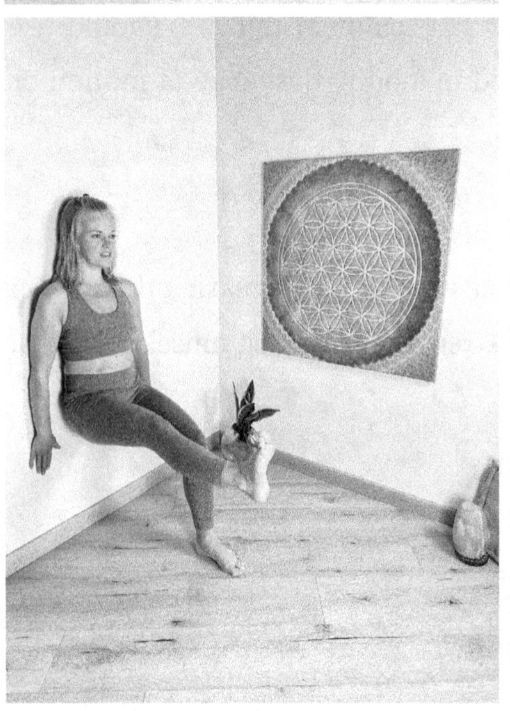

Step-by-Step Instructions:

1. **Starting Position:** Stand with your back against a sturdy wall, ensuring that your entire back and glutes are in contact with the wall. Take a step to the side, positioning your feet slightly more than shoulder-width apart. Turn your feet out slightly to achieve a comfortable stance.

2. **Descending Phase:** Breathe in deeply and slowly slide your body down the wall, bending your knees at a 90-degree angle. Your thighs should be parallel to the floor, and your weight should be supported by the wall. Bring your arms down straight against the wall, with your palms flat for added support.

3. **Leg Extension:** Lift your right leg off the floor, extending it straight out in front of you. Keep your foot flexed and parallel to the ground. Hold this position for 5 seconds, focusing on engaging your quadriceps and maintaining stability throughout your core.

4. **Return to Starting Position:** Gently lower your right leg back to the floor and stand up, allowing a brief rest period of 30 seconds before repeating the exercise.

5. **Repeat with Left Leg:** Take a step to the side and slide down the wall into the squat position again. Lift

your left leg off the floor, extending it straight in front of you. Hold for 5 seconds, emphasizing control and balance.

6. **Complete Repetitions:** Alternate between lifting your right and left legs, completing a full repetition of the alternating leg extension exercise. Aim to perform 10 repetitions on each leg, maintaining proper form and control throughout.

Warnings and Contraindications:

- Avoid allowing your knees to extend beyond your toes during the wall sit phase of the exercise. This can place excessive strain on the knee joints and increase the risk of injury.
- Individuals with pre-existing knee or hip injuries should exercise caution when performing the Wall Sit with Alternating Leg Extension. Consider consulting with a physical therapist for personalized modifications or alternative exercises.

Advanced Version:

- **Increase in leg extension time:** Extend the time for holding the raised leg to 10 seconds. This exercise advancement enhances the strengthening of the muscles in the lower body.

24 Wall Sit Calf Raises

Affected Area: Legs and buttocks.

Objectives of the Exercise: Wall Sit Calf Raises combine the advantages of wall sits and calf raises to target and strengthen the muscles in the lower body, especially the calves, thighs, hamstrings, and glutes. This exercise aims to improve lower body strength, endurance, and muscle tone. By incorporating the support of the wall, it provides added stability and allows for proper form while performing calf raises. The controlled up-and-down movement engages multiple muscle groups concurrently, offering a comprehensive lower body workout.

Step-by-Step Instructions:

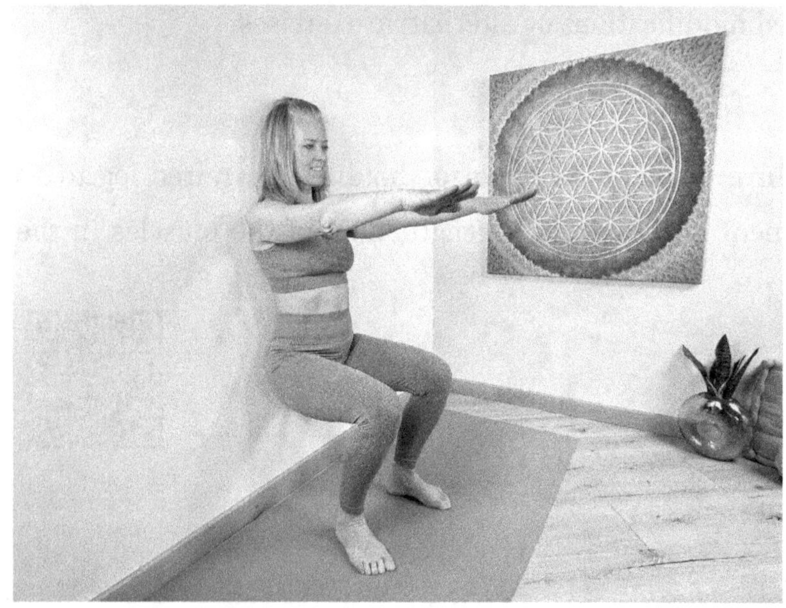

1. **Starting Position:** Stand with your back against a sturdy wall, ensuring that your entire back and glutes are in contact with the wall. Take a step to the side, allowing your legs to be slightly more than shoulder-width apart. Turn your feet out slightly to establish a comfortable stance.

2. **Descending Phase:** Breathe in deeply and slowly slide your body down the wall, bending your knees at a 90-degree angle. Your thighs should be parallel to the floor, and your weight should be supported by the wall. Bring your arms out straight in front of you at chest height, with your palms facing the floor. This position sets the foundation for the wall sit.

3. **Calf Raise:** Move into the calf raise by transferring your body weight onto the balls of your feet. Propel

through the balls of your feet, lifting your heels as high as possible, and contract your calf muscles at the top of the movement. Hold this raised position for two seconds, focusing on the contraction in your calf muscles.

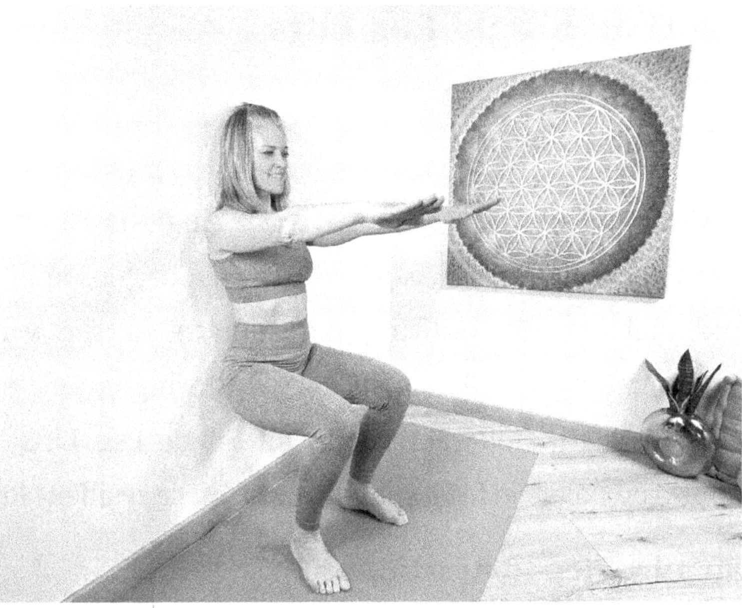

4. **Return to Starting Position:** Gradually lower your heels back to the floor over a two-second period, returning to the flat foot position. Control the descent to engage the muscles and maximize the effectiveness of the exercise.

5. **Repetitions:** Perform the ball-to-flat foot movement for 10 repetitions initially, gradually increasing the number of repetitions as you build strength and endurance. Aim to work your way up to 20 repetitions, maintaining a steady pace and focusing on the quality of each movement.

Warnings and Contraindications:

- Avoid locking your knees at the top of the calf raise movement to prevent strain on the joints.
- Individuals with knee or ankle injuries or conditions such as arthritis should use caution when performing Wall Sit Calf Raises. Commence with a smaller range of motion and incrementally enhance it as strength and mobility advance.

Advanced Version:

Single-Leg Wall Sit Calf Raises: Lift one foot off the ground and perform the calf raises with the other leg, maintaining the wall sit position with the supporting leg. This variation challenges your balance and stability while intensifying the engagement of the calf muscles.

25 Wall Single-Leg Lifts

Affected Area: Legs and buttocks.

Objectives of the Exercise: Wall Single-Leg Lifts are a targeted Pilates exercise aimed at strengthening the legs, especially the quadriceps and hamstrings, while also enhancing balance and stability. By utilizing the support of the wall, this exercise provides a controlled environment for isolating each leg, fostering muscle engagement, and promoting overall lower body strength. Incorporating Wall Single-Leg Lifts into your Pilates routine contributes to improved balance, leg strength, and a more resilient lower body.

Step-by-Step Instructions:

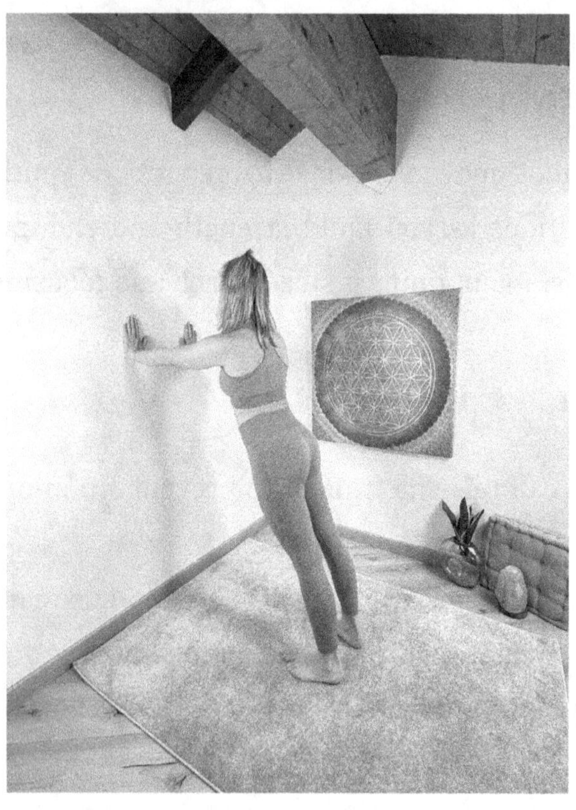
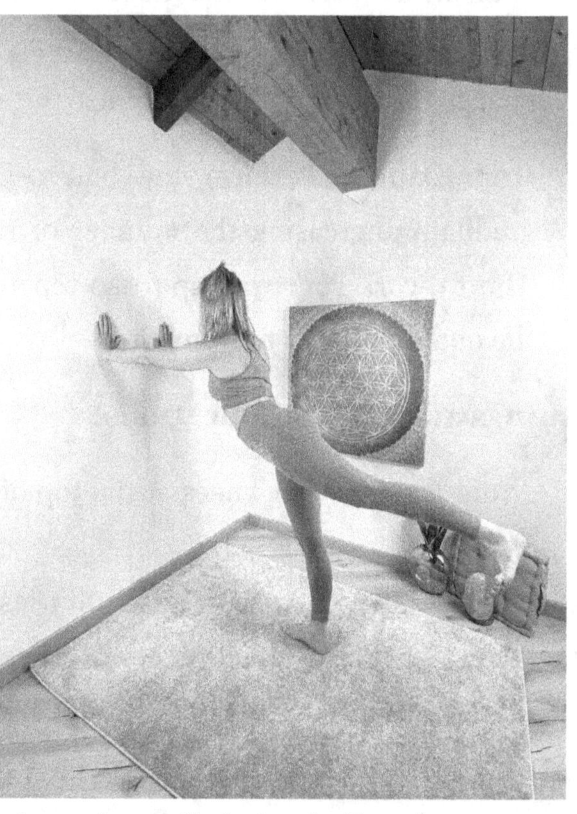

1. **Starting Position:** Stand a few feet away from the wall, facing it directly. Ensure your feet are hip-width apart, creating a stable base. Position your hands lightly against the wall for support and balance.

2. **Lifting Motion:** Choose one leg to lift off the ground, extending it straight and parallel to the floor. This lifting motion engages the quadriceps, hamstrings, and calf muscles. The hands on the wall provide stability during this phase.

3. **Stability and Balance:** Maintain the lifted leg position for a few seconds, focusing on stability and balance. This phase emphasizes the activation of the supporting leg's muscles and challenges the core to contribute to overall body stability.

4. **Lowering Phase:** Gently lower the lifted leg back to the starting position, controlling the descent. This controlled movement helps in targeting specific muscle groups while minimizing momentum.

5. **Repeat with Opposite Leg:** After completing the repetitions with one leg, replicate the same movement pattern with the opposite leg. Lift the second leg, hold for a few seconds, and then gently lower it back to the starting position.

6. **Repetitions and Sets:** Aim to complete 3 sets of 10-12 repetitions for each leg. This repetition range ensures a comprehensive workout for the legs, promoting strength and stability.

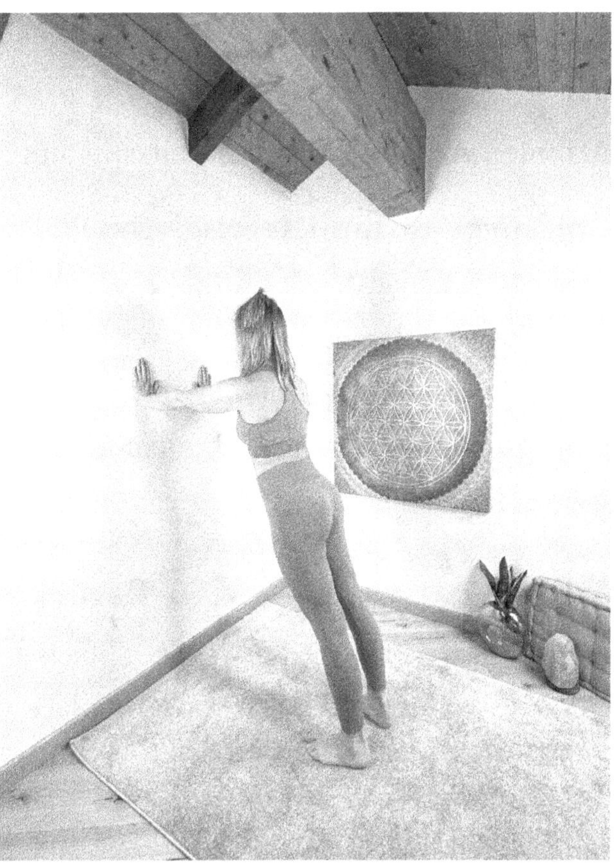

Warnings and Contraindications:

- Individuals with knee, ankle, or hip injuries should exercise caution when performing Wall Single-Leg Lifts. Commence with a smaller range of motion and gradually increase as strength and mobility improve.
- Avoid locking the supporting knee during the lifting phase to prevent strain or injury. Keep a slight bend in the knee to maintain joint integrity and stability.

Advanced Version:

- **Single-Leg Squat Variation:** Instead of simply lifting the leg, perform a single-leg squat with the supporting leg while keeping the lifted leg extended. This variation introduces a dynamic component to the exercise, effectively targeting additional muscle groups and augmenting overall lower body strength and stability.

26 Wall-Supported Dynamic Back Lunge

Affected Area: Legs, glutes, and core muscles

Objectives of the Exercise: The Wall-Supported Dynamic Back Lunge is a lower body exercise designed to target the legs, glutes, and core muscles. The primary objectives of this exercise are to strengthen the lower body muscles, improve balance and stability, and enhance overall lower body function. By incorporating the wall for support, it also helps in maintaining proper form and alignment throughout the movement.

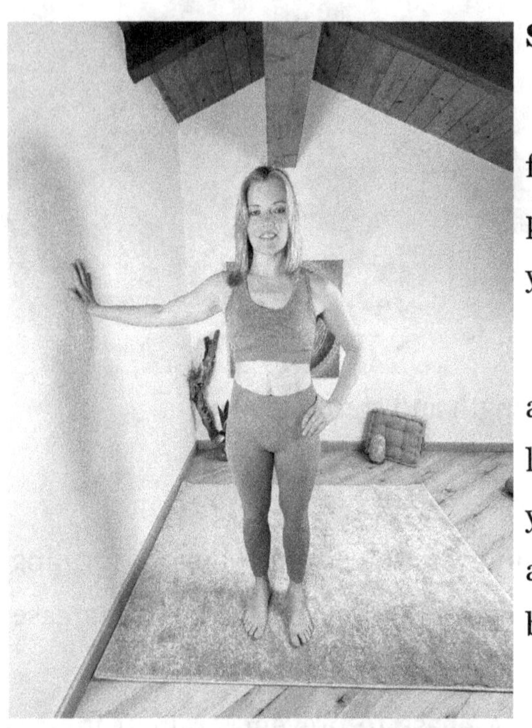

Step-by-Step Instructions:

1. **Starting Position:** Stand with your right side facing the wall. Extend your left arm out straight and place your right hand, palm flat against the wall. Keep your feet hip-width apart and parallel to each other.

2. **Exhale and Step Back:** Breathe in deeply and as you breathe out, take a good step back with your left leg. The left foot should land far enough back that when you lower into the lunge, both knees are bent at approximately 90-degree angles. Ensure your feet are both facing forward in a straight line.

3. **Lower into Lunge:** Lower your body straight down by bending both knees, keeping your weight primarily on the front leg. Your right knee should be directly above your ankle, and your left knee should hover just above the ground.

4. **Drive Knee Up:** As you begin to return to the starting position, push through the heel of your right foot and drive your left knee up to a 90-degree angle in front of you. This movement should resemble an exaggerated march, engaging your core for balance.

5. **Repeat with left Leg:** Complete 10 repetitions with your left leg stepping back. Focus on maintaining a smooth, controlled movement throughout the exercise.

Keep your core engaged and avoid leaning too far forward or backward.

6. **Switch to Opposite Side:** Now, stand with your left side facing the wall. Repeat the same steps with your right leg, taking a good step back with your right leg this time. Lower into a lunge, ensuring both knees are bent at 90-degree angles, and then drive your right knee up as you return to the starting position.

7. **Complete 10 Repetitions:** Perform 10 repetitions with your right leg stepping back. Focus on the quality of each movement, maintaining proper form, and engaging the muscles of the legs and core throughout.

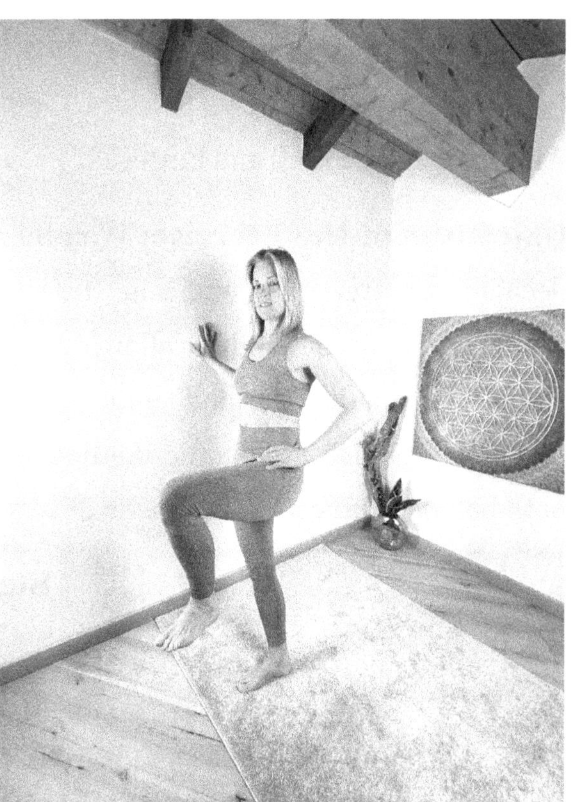

8. **Breathing:** Breathe in deeply as you step back into the lunge position, breathe out as you push back up to the starting position, and continue to breathe steadily throughout the exercise. The breathing should be controlled and coordinated with each movement.

9. **Repeat Sets:** Depending on your fitness level, aim to complete 2-3 sets of 10 repetitions on each leg. Allow for a brief rest period between sets to recover and maintain proper form.

Warnings and Contraindications:

- If you have any knee, hip, or ankle injuries, exercise caution when performing the Wall-Supported Dynamic Back Lunge. Start with a smaller range of motion and gradually increase it as your strength and mobility improve.
- Individuals with balance issues or who are new to exercise should begin with a shallower lunge and focus on stability.

Advanced Version:

- **Pulse Lunges:** After lowering into the lunge position, instead of returning to the starting position immediately, perform a small pulsing motion by moving up and down within a short range. This continuous tension on the muscles increases the burn and helps improve muscle endurance.

27 Wall-Supported Side Kicks

Affected Area: Legs and buttocks.

Objectives of the Exercise: Wall-Supported Side Kicks are a targeted lower body exercise designed to strengthen and tone the legs and buttocks. By utilizing the support of a wall, this exercise enhances stability, allowing for controlled side kicks that primarily engage the hip abductors, quadriceps, and glutes. Integrating Wall-Supported Side Kicks into your fitness regimen provides a dynamic method for sculpting and fortifying the lower body, enhancing both balance and coordination.

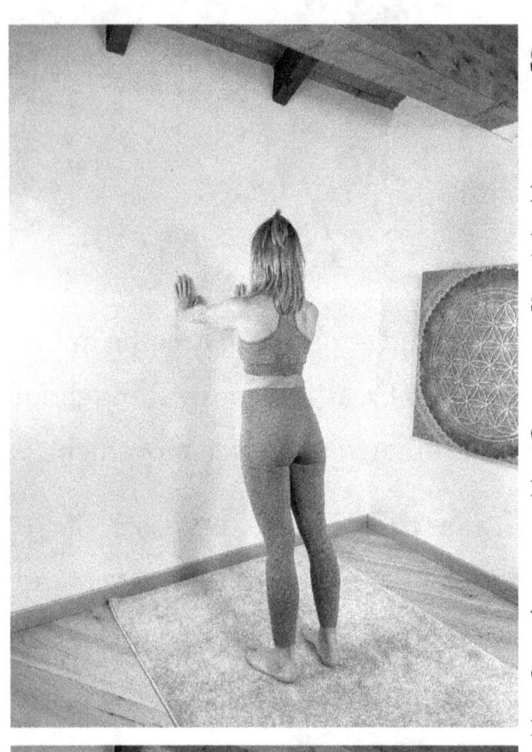

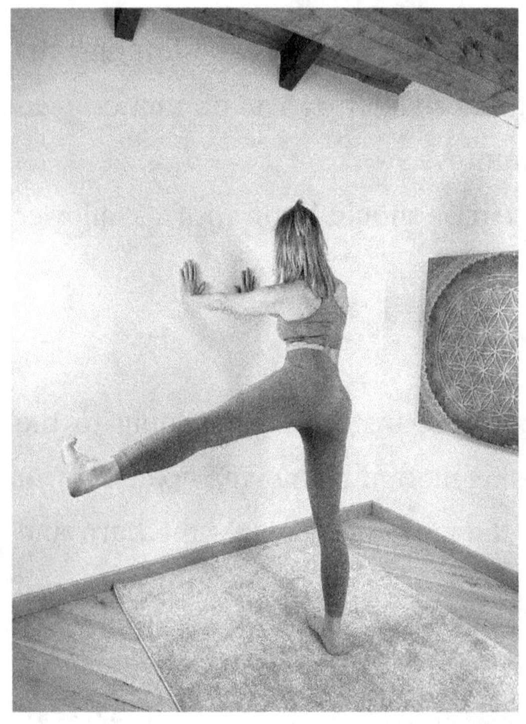

Step-by-Step Instructions:

1. **Starting Position:** Stand in front of a wall, maintaining a distance of approximately an arm's length. Put your hands against the wall at shoulder height for support.

2. **Lift One Leg:** Lift one leg off the ground, extending it out to the side. Ensure that your knee remains straight during this motion.

3. **Execute Side Kick:** Swing your extended leg out to the side, aiming to reach hip level or higher. Focus on engaging the hip abductors and maintaining a controlled movement.

4. **Engage Core:** Keep your core tight throughout the exercise to enhance stability and control. A stable core contributes to better balance and effective muscle engagement.

5. **Return to Starting Position:** Bring your leg back to the initial starting position in a controlled manner. Avoid abrupt movements to maximize muscle engagement.

6. **Repeat:** Aim to perform 10-12 repetitions on each leg for 2-3 sets, depending on your fitness level and goals.

7. **Switch Legs:** Shift to the other leg and repeat the side kicks, ensuring symmetry and balanced engagement of both lower limbs.

Warnings and Contraindications:

- Individuals with knee, hip, or lower back issues should exercise caution when performing Wall-Supported Side Kicks. Commence with a smaller range of motion and gradually increase as strength and flexibility improve.
- Avoid jerky or uncontrolled movements, as this can increase the risk of injury. Focus on executing each side kick with precision and control.

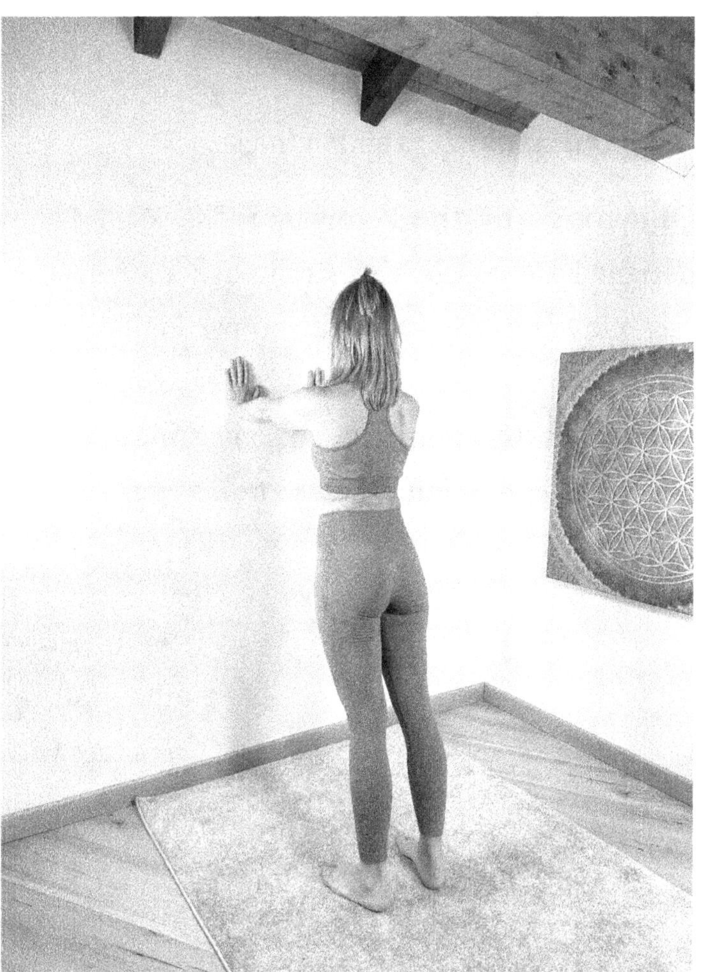

Advanced Version:

- **Pulse Movement:** Instead of completing a full range of motion with each side kick, incorporate pulse movements at the top of the kick. Lift your leg to hip level and pulse it up and down slightly before returning to the starting position. This variation increases time under tension and maximizes muscle activation.

28 Wall Lateral Squat

Affected Area: Legs and buttocks.

Objectives of the Exercise: The Wall Lateral Squat is a targeted lower body exercise designed to engage and strengthen the muscles of the legs and buttocks while promoting flexibility and balance. By incorporating lateral movement into a traditional squat and utilizing the support of the wall, this exercise challenges different muscle groups and enhances overall lower body function. The objectives include improving leg strength, enhancing hip mobility, and promoting stability and coordination.

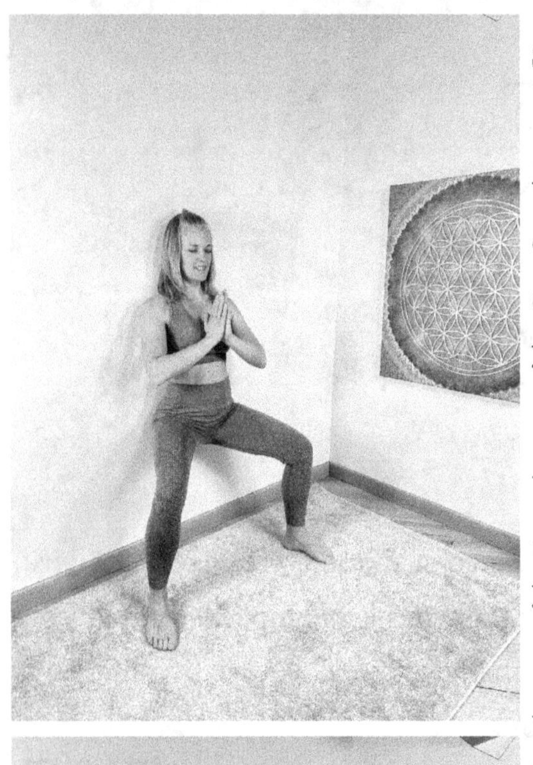

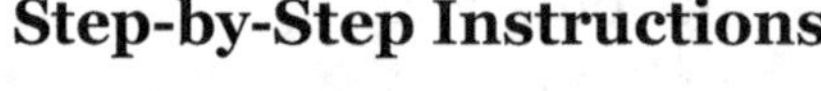

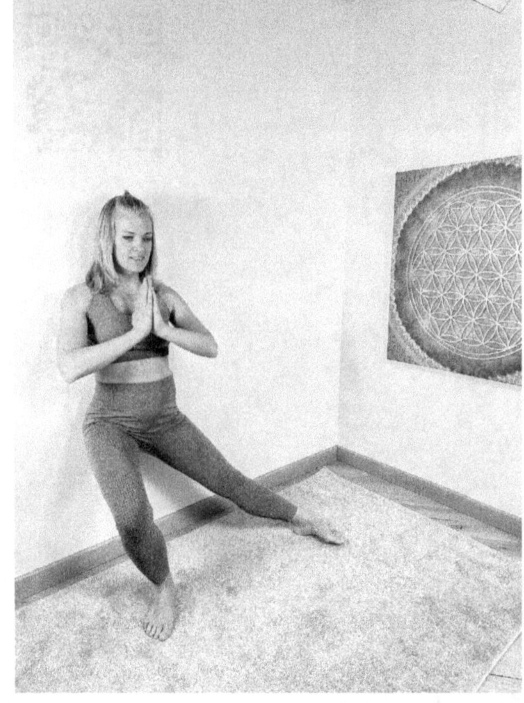

Step-by-Step Instructions:

1. **Starting Position:** Stand with your back against the wall, ensuring your entire back and glutes are in contact with the wall. Take a step to the side, creating a stance slightly wider than shoulder-width apart. Turn your feet slightly outward.

2. **Descending into Squat:** Breathe in and begin to lower your body down the wall, bending your knees at a 90-degree angle. Allow the wall to provide support as you descend into a squat position.

3. **Initiate Lateral Movement:** Push off the wall with your right foot, moving towards the right side. Ensure that your knees are aligned with your toes during the lateral squat.

4. **Maintain Control:** As you squat laterally, maintain control and aim for a comfortable depth. The supporting wall allows for controlled movement, enabling you to focus on engaging the muscles of the inner and outer thighs.

5. **Return to Center:** Push through your left foot to return to the center, aligning your body with the wall. Ensure that both feet are flat on the ground and your back is still in contact with the wall.

6. **Repeat on Opposite Side:** Perform the lateral squat in the opposite direction, pushing off the wall with your left foot this time. Maintain proper form and controlled movements.

7. **Repetitions:** Aim for 3 sets of 12-15 repetitions on each side, adjusting the intensity based on your fitness level. Focus on the quality of each movement to maximize effectiveness.

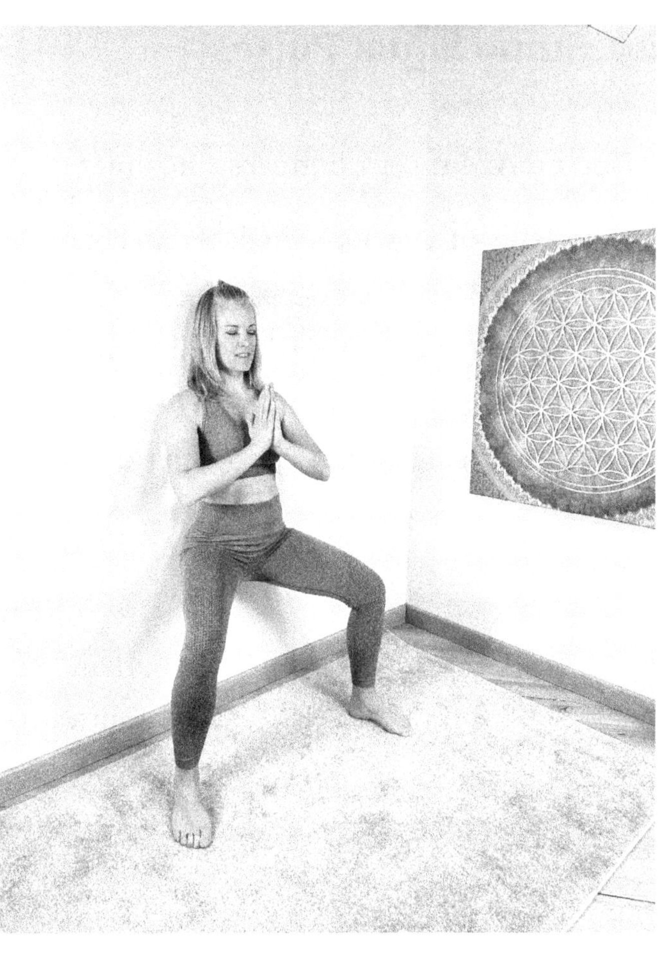

Warnings and Contraindications:

- Individuals with knee, hip, or lower back issues should exercise caution when performing the Wall Lateral Squat. Commence with a smaller range of motion and gradually increase as strength and flexibility improve.

- Avoid leaning too far forward or allowing the knees to extend past the toes during the squatting motion, as this can place undue stress on the joints.

Advanced Version:

To advance the Wall Lateral Squat and further challenge your lower body muscles, you can incorporate the following modifications:

- **Pulsing Motion:** At the bottom of the squat, add a pulsing motion by performing small, controlled pulses up and down to increase time under tension and maximize muscle activation.

29 Sumo Squat Pulses

Affected Area: Legs, buttocks, and inner thighs.

Objectives of the Exercise: Sumo squat pulses, particularly when adapted for the wall in Pilates, target the quadriceps, glutes, and inner thighs. This exercise aims to strengthen and tone these muscle groups while improving lower body endurance and stability. By utilizing the support of a wall, proper form can be maintained, allowing for maximum engagement of the leg muscles and reducing the risk of injury.

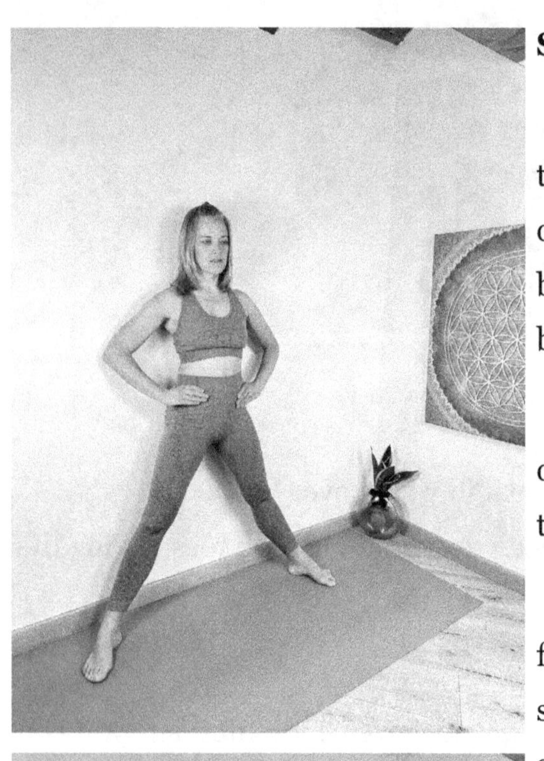

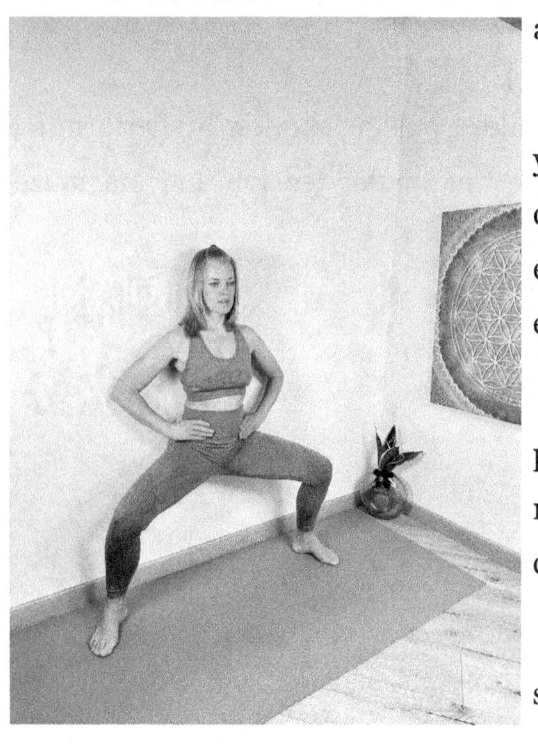

Step-by-Step Instructions:

1. **Starting Position:** Stand with your feet wider than shoulder-width apart, toes pointing slightly outward. Position yourself facing a wall, ensuring your back remains straight, and your lower back is supported by the wall.

2. **Hand Placement:** Put your hands on your hips or hold onto the wall for balance and support throughout the exercise.

3. **Descending into the Squat:** Descend by flexing your knees and hips, simulating the motion of sitting into an unseen chair. Ensure that your knees are aligned over your toes without extending beyond them.

4. **Squat Depth:** Strive to reach a position where your thighs are parallel to the floor while maintaining contact with the wall behind you. This ensures proper engagement of the leg muscles and maximizes the effectiveness of the exercise.

5. **Initiating the Pulses:** Once in the squat position, begin pulsing up and down in a small range of motion. Move about an inch up and down, keeping constant tension in your leg muscles.

6. **Breathing:** Breathe in as you lower into the squat position, and breathe out as you pulse up and

down, maintaining the movement. Focus on controlled breathing to synchronize with the pulsing motion.

7. **Repetitions and Sets:** Start with 10-15 pulses for one set, and aim to complete 2-3 sets, then gradually increase the number of reps and sets as you become more comfortable with the exercise.

Warnings and Contraindications:

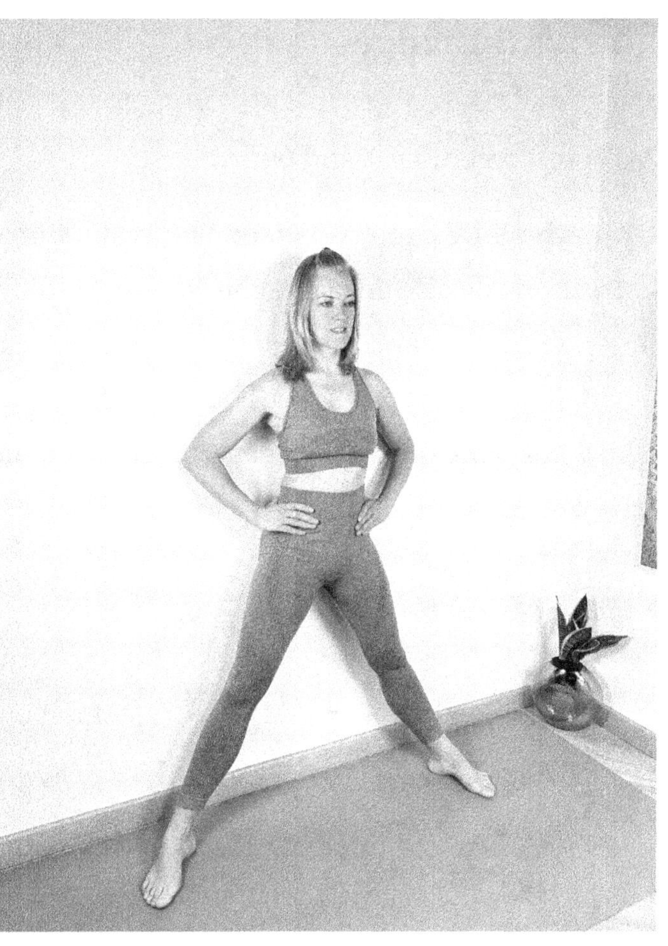

- Maintain proper form to avoid straining the lower back and knees. Refrain from rounding the back or allowing the knees to extend beyond the toes.
- If you feel any kind of discomfort or pain, you should instantly stop what you're doing and reevaluate your form. To prevent pushing through pain, it is crucial to pay attention to what your body is telling you.

Advanced Version:

- **Increase Repetitions:** Gradually increase the number of pulses per set or the number of sets performed to further challenge your muscles and improve endurance. Strive to push your limits while maintaining proper form and technique.

30 Wall Bridge

Affected Area: Legs and buttocks.

Objectives of the Exercise: The Wall Bridge targets and tones the muscles of the legs and buttocks while also engaging the core for stability and support. This exercise aims to strengthen the posterior chain, including the glutes and lower back, leading to improved strength, flexibility, and overall lower body function. By utilizing the wall for support, the Wall Bridge allows for controlled movement and precise muscle activation, enhancing the effectiveness of the exercise.

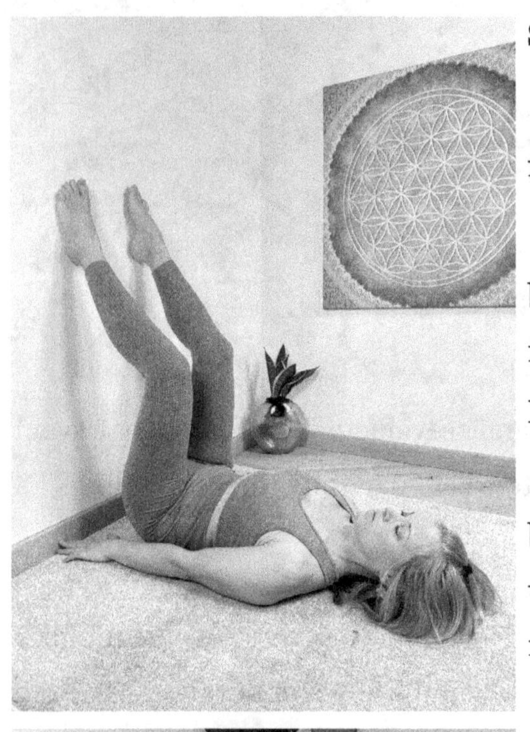

Step-by-Step Instructions:

1. **Starting Position:** Lie on your back with your feet flat on the ground, spaced hip-width apart.

2. **Core Engagement:** Gently press your lower back onto the ground, engaging your core muscles. This initial step is crucial for maintaining proper form and preventing unnecessary strain on the lower back.

3. **Hip Lift:** Gradually lift your hips off the ground by pushing through your heels and upper back against the wall. Focus on the activation of your glutes and maintain core engagement throughout this movement.

4. **Alignment Focus:** Elevate your hips 'til your body forms a straight line from your shoulders to your knees. Pay close attention to proper alignment, ensuring that your head, shoulders, and hips are in a straight line.

5. **Hold Position:** Maintain the raised position for a few seconds, concentrating on the engagement in your glutes and lower back. Avoid overextending your lower back during this phase, emphasizing controlled movement.

6. **Lowering Phase:** Lower your hips back down to the starting position in a deliberate manner. Continue to engage your core to control the descent.

7. **Repetitions:** Perform 3 sets of 12-15 repetitions, focusing on the quality of each movement rather than quantity. This repetition range ensures optimal muscle engagement and endurance.

Warnings and Contraindications:

- Refrain from excessive arching of your lower back throughout the exercise to prevent potential strain or injury. Concentrate on maintaining a neutral spine position by activating your core muscles.
- If you have pre-existing lower back issues or injuries, exercise caution when executing the Wall Bridge. Commence with a limited range of motion and progressively expand it as strength and flexibility enhance.

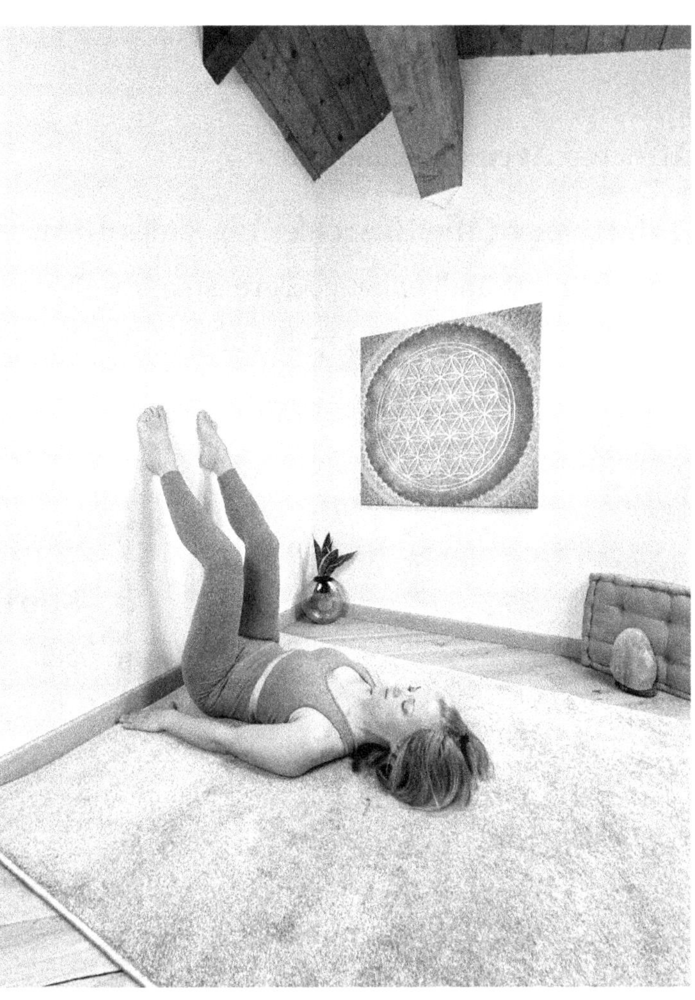

Advanced Version:

- **Single-Leg Wall Bridge:** Lift one foot off the ground and perform the bridge exercise with only one leg. This variation increases the demand on the stabilizing muscles of the hips and core, enhancing balance and strength.

31 Leg Slides

Affected Area: Legs and core.

Objectives of the Exercise: Leg Slides are designed to strengthen the leg muscles, improve hip mobility, and enhance core stability. This exercise effectively targets the hamstrings, quadriceps, glutes, and hip flexors, while also engaging the deep core muscles. The smooth sliding motion involves multiple muscle groups, making it a valuable inclusion in your workout regimen.

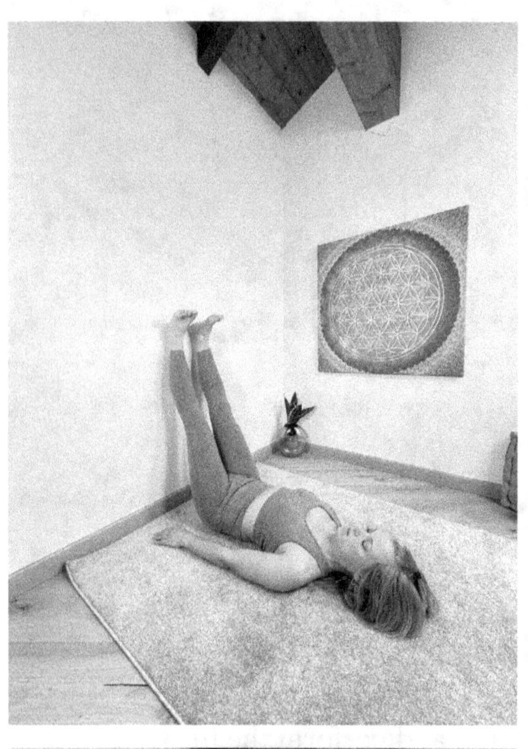

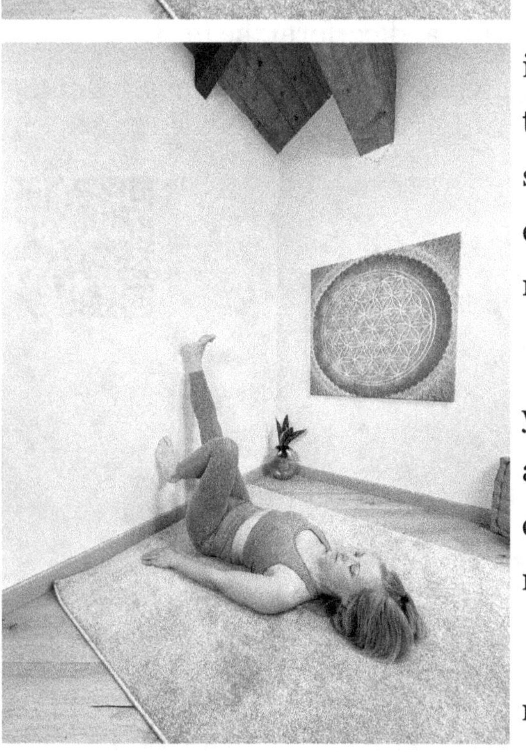

Step-by-Step Instructions:

1. **Starting Position:** Commence by lying flat on your back, either on an exercise mat or a comfortable surface.Extend your legs completely, leaning them against the wall, and let your arms rest naturally at your sides. Ensure your spine is in a neutral position with a slight natural curve in the lower back.

2. **Engage Core Muscles:** Gently pull your navel toward your spine to engage your core muscles. This action helps stabilize your spine and pelvis, preparing your body for the movement.

3. **Slide One Leg Away:** As you breathe out, initiate a deliberate slide of one leg. Keep the leg close to the floor, bending the knee completely, maintaining a straight alignment from the hip to the toes. Focus on engaging the leg muscles as you perform the sliding motion.

4. **Return to the starting position:** Breathe in as you skillfully bring the leg back to the starting position, aligning it with the other leg. Ensure a smooth and controlled movement during the return phase to maximize muscle engagement.

5. **Repeat with Opposite Leg:** Exhale and replicate the movement with the opposite leg. Ensure

proper form and alignment are maintained throughout the exercise, emphasizing movement quality rather than speed.

6. **Alternate Legs:** Continue with the alternating rhythm of leg slides. Aim for a steady and controlled pace, maintaining core engagement to stabilize the pelvis and spine.

7. **Complete Repetitions:** Perform 10-12 repetitions on each leg, alternating between the left and right sides.

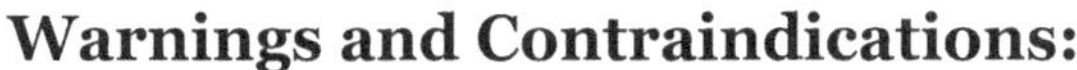

Warnings and Contraindications:

- Avoid overextending the legs or arching the lower back during the movement. Keep the range of motion within a comfortable and controlled range to prevent strain or injury.
- If you have any existing knee conditions or injuries, consult with a healthcare professional prior to performing Leg Slides to ensure it is safe for your specific condition.

Advanced Version:

- **Slide both legs:** starting from the same position, slide both legs against the wall, and additionally, keeping your hands behind your head, raise your shoulder blades and bring your head towards your knees. Thus, performing an abdominal crunch. Perform 20 repetitions.

32 Quadruped Leg Extension

Affected Area: Legs, buttocks, and core.

Objectives of the Exercise: The Quadruped Leg Extension targets and strengthens the muscles of the legs, buttocks, and core while promoting stability and balance. This exercise aims to improve lower body strength, enhance muscle endurance, and increase overall core stability. By incorporating the support of a wall, the exercise offers added resistance and challenges various muscle groups, making it an effective addition to any workout routine.

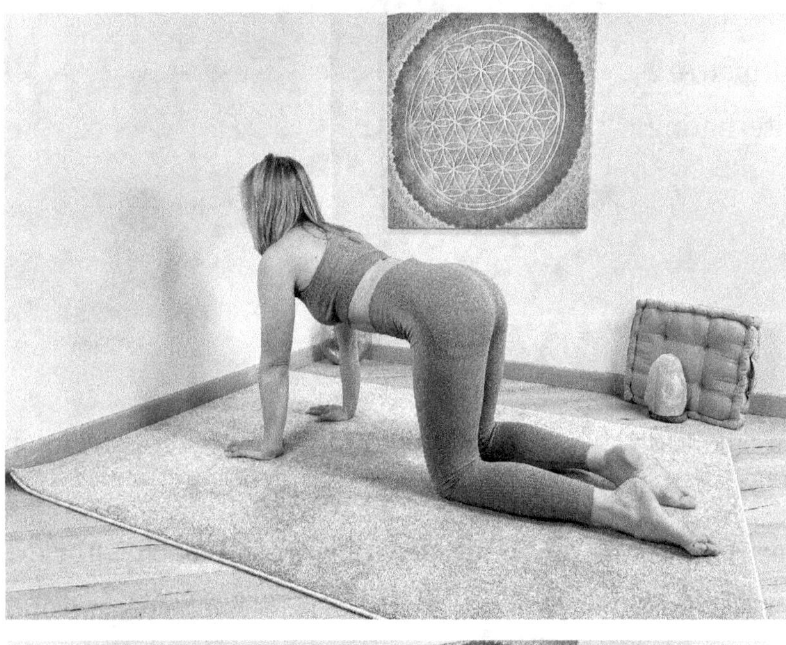

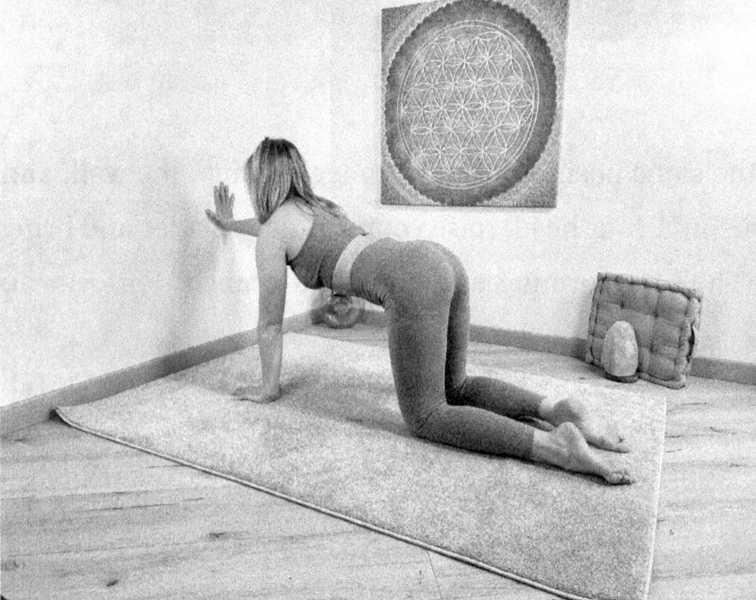

Step-by-Step Instructions:

1. **Starting Position:** Stand facing the wall and position yourself on all fours, ensuring your wrists are aligned directly under your shoulders and the knees are beneath your hips. Keep a neutral spine with a flat back and engage your core muscles for stability.

2. **Arm Placement:** Elevate your right arm to shoulder height, pressing your right palm firmly against the wall. Retract your right shoulder blade downward and backward to enhance stability. Find a distance from the wall that allows for elbow extension while ensuring a secure wall contact.

3. **Leg Extension:** Extend your left leg behind you, pointing your toes away from the body. Gradually elevate your left leg to hip level or higher, focusing on maintaining a level pelvis throughout the movement. Lower the leg until your toes hover just an inch or two above the ground, ensuring controlled movements.

4. **Repetitions:** Execute 10 repetitions on one side before switching to the opposite side. This ensures balanced muscle engagement and development, targeting both the left and right sides of the body.

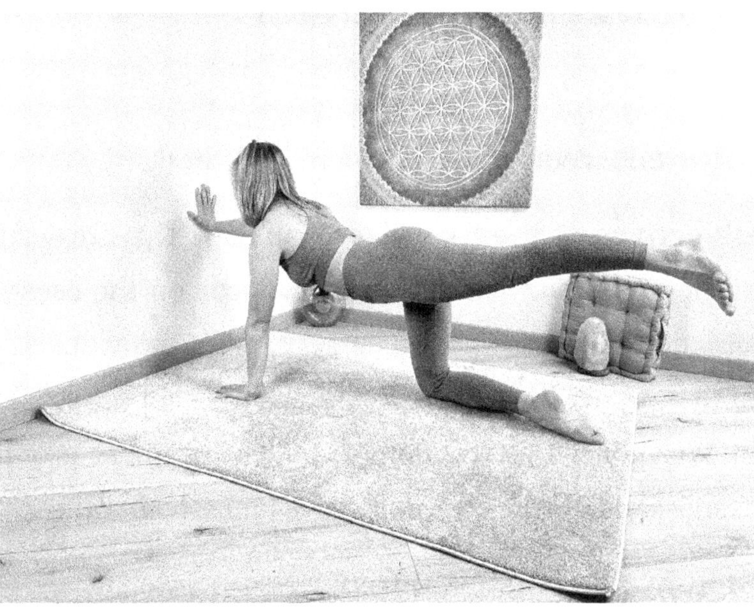

Warnings and Contraindications:

- Individuals with wrist or shoulder injuries should use caution when performing the Quadruped Leg Extension. Ensure that the wrists are properly supported and avoid placing excessive strain on the shoulders.
- Avoid overarching or rounding the back during the movement. Maintain a neutral spine position to prevent strain on the lower back and ensure proper alignment.

Advanced Version:

Knee raise: In order to make the challenge more difficult, curl your right toes under while simultaneously lifting your right knee off the ground. Do the leg extensions while holding this hovering position, engaging both core and leg muscles simultaneously. This variation adds an additional layer of difficulty, elevating the overall effectiveness of the exercise.

Affected Area: Arms, shoulders, and chest.

Objectives of the Exercise: Wall Push-Ups are designed to strengthen and tone the muscles of the upper body, with a primary focus on the chest, shoulders, and triceps. This accessible variation serves as an ideal entry point for individuals seeking to cultivate strength and stability in their upper body while leveraging the supportive framework provided by a wall. By engaging in Wall Push-Ups, beginners can lay a robust groundwork for more advanced bodyweight exercises, fostering comprehensive upper body fitness.

Step-by-Step Instructions:

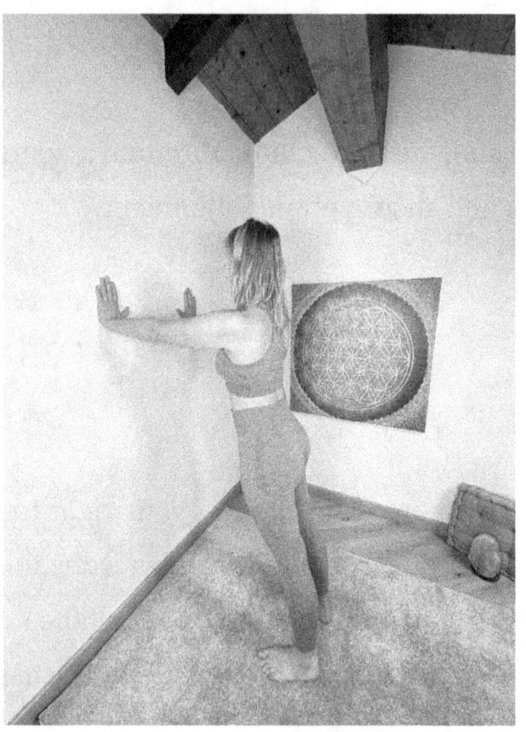
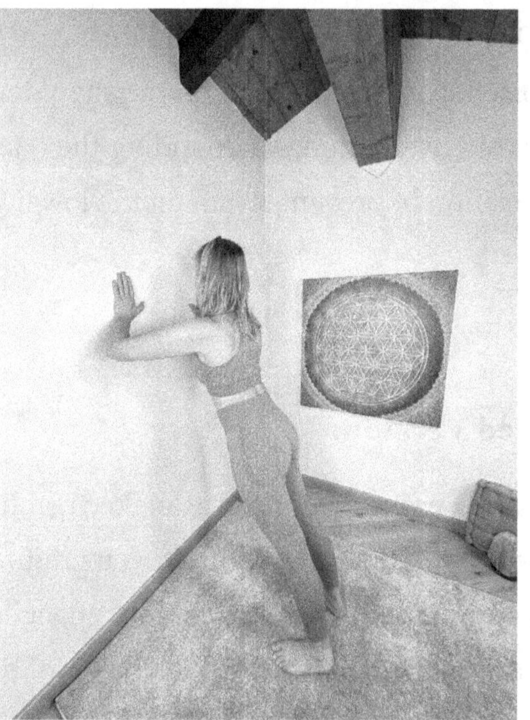

1. **Starting Position:** Stand in front of a wall with your feet positioned hip-width apart to establish a stable base. Arrange your hands so that they are a little wider than shoulder-width apart and rest them on the wall at shoulder height. In order to keep a straight alignment from your head to your heels, you should make sure that your core is engaged. This will provide you with stability and support.

2. **Initiate the Movement:** Begin the exercise by bending your elbows and gradually lowering your chest towards the wall. Maintain a straight line by keeping your body in a straight line during the exercise. Refrain from arching your back or drooping your back. Concentrate on preserving proper form and control as you descend your body towards the wall.

3. **Breathing Technique:** Exhale as you exert force, pushing back to the initial position by fully extending your arms. Breathe in as you lower your body towards the wall, and breathe out as you push back up. Focus on breathing rhythmically and maintaining a steady pace throughout the exercise.

4. **Repetition Range:** Aim to complete 12 to 15 repetitions of Wall Push-Ups, focusing on quality over quantity. Ensure that each repetition is performed with proper form, controlled movement, and deliberate engagement of the targeted muscles – chest, shoulders, and triceps.

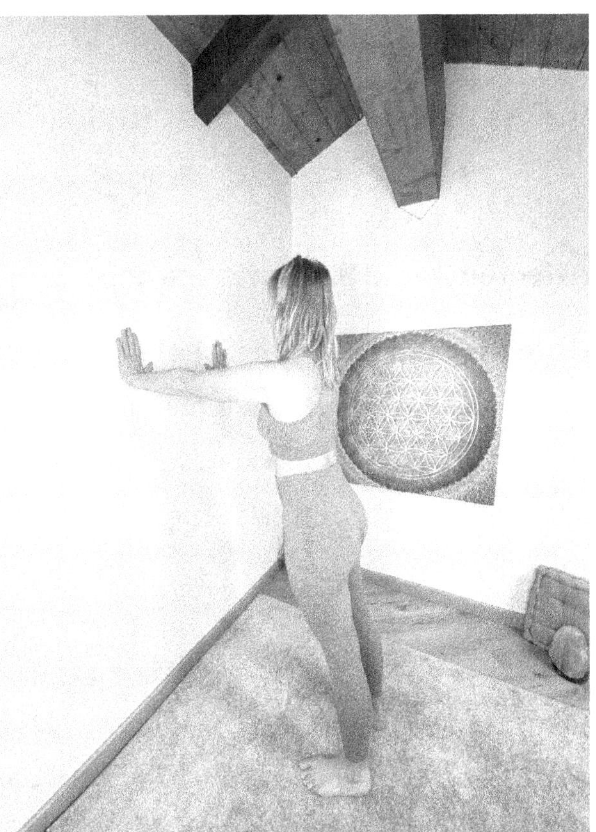

5. **Finishing Position:** Return to the starting position with your arms fully extended, pushing away from the wall with force. Maintain a straight alignment of your body and engage your core muscles for stability.

Warnings and Contraindications:

- Prevent overarching or rounding of the back during Wall Push-Ups to mitigate strain or injury to the spine. Concentrate on maintaining a neutral spine position and engaging your core muscles throughout the exercise.
- If you have any pre-existing medical conditions or physical limitations that may impact your ability to safely perform Wall Push-Ups, consult with a healthcare provider before attempting this exercise.

Advanced Version:

- **Leg raise**: before performing the wall squat, raise your left leg and then perform the squat, then alternate the raised leg and repeat the wall squat. Perform 20 repetitions.

34 Wall Shoulder Shrugs

Affected Area: Shoulders and upper arms.

Objectives of the Exercise: Wall Shoulder Shrugs aim to strengthen and tone the muscles of the shoulders, primarily targeting the deltoids and trapezius muscles. By incorporating the support of a wall, this exercise provides stability and control, allowing individuals to focus on proper form and muscle engagement. The primary objectives include enhancing shoulder stability, improving posture, and fortifying the upper body.

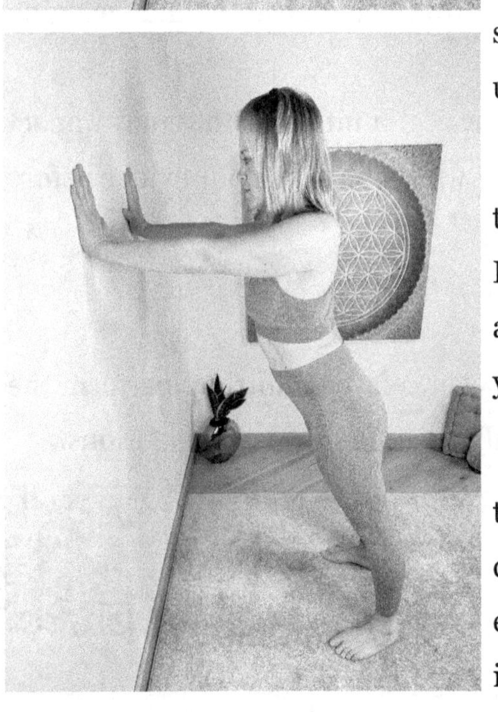

Step-by-Step Instructions:

1. **Starting Position:** Put your feet shoulder-width apart and stand in front of the wall that is facing you. Take a position where your palms are against the wall at shoulder height, and make sure that your arms are fully stretched out. To maintain stability, make sure that your body is in a straight line from head to toe and that your core muscles are engaged.

2. **Core Engagement:** Tighten your core muscles to establish a stable base. This core engagement will help support your body throughout the exercise and prevent unnecessary strain on the lower back.

3. **Shoulder Elevation:** Elevate your shoulders toward your ears, engaging the upper trapezius muscles. Focus on a controlled and deliberate upward movement, avoiding any jerky motions. Keep your arms straight and your palms pressed firmly against the wall.

4. **Hold and Contract:** At the top of the shrug, hold the position for a brief moment. Focus on feeling the contraction in your shoulder muscles as they work to elevate your shoulders towards your ears. Maintain tension in the muscles without locking your elbows or hyperextending your shoulders.

5. **Lowering Phase:** Lower your shoulders back down in a controlled manner, gradually releasing the tension in your shoulder muscles. Avoid letting your shoulders drop suddenly or collapsing into the movement. Emphasize a smooth and controlled descent to maximize the effectiveness of the exercise.

6. **Repetition Range:** Perform 12-15 repetitions of the shoulder shrugs, with the emphasis being placed on the quality of the movement instead of its speed. Ensure that each repetition is performed with proper form and controlled movement. Pay attention to the activation of the shoulder muscles throughout the entire range of motion.

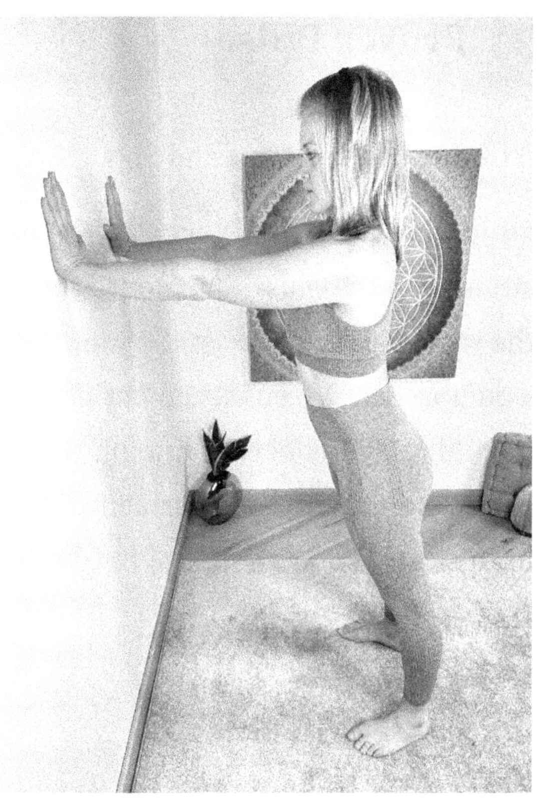

7. **Rest and Sets:** Allow a brief rest period between sets to recover before performing the next set of shoulder shrugs. Aim to complete 3 sets of Wall Shoulder Shrugs for a comprehensive shoulder workout, gradually increasing the intensity and resistance as you progress.

Warnings and Contraindications:

- Avoid shrugging your shoulders excessively or using momentum to lift the weight. Focus on controlled movements and proper form to prevent strain or injury to the shoulder muscles.

- Before attempting Wall Shoulder Shrugs, should you have any already present illnesses, it is highly recommended that you seek the advice of a healthcare expert first or if you have physical limitations that could impact your ability to perform the exercise safely.

Advanced Version:

- **Single-Arm Wall Shoulder Shrugs:** Perform the shoulder shrugs with one arm at a time, alternating between left and right shoulders. This unilateral variation helps correct muscle imbalances and improves overall shoulder stability.

35 Prayer Pulse

Affected Area: Arms and Shoulders.

Objectives of the Exercise: The Prayer Pulse exercise is specifically crafted to activate and strengthen the muscles in your arms and shoulders. Its rhythmic pulsing motion, coupled with the seated stance against the wall, introduces a distinctive element to this workout, promoting a comprehensive enhancement of upper body strength. By integrating mindfulness into your breathing and concentrating on the deliberate pulses, you not only sculpt your arms but also enrich your mind-body harmony. This routine proves especially advantageous for those aiming to cultivate sleek and well-defined arm and shoulder muscles.

Step-by-Step Instructions:

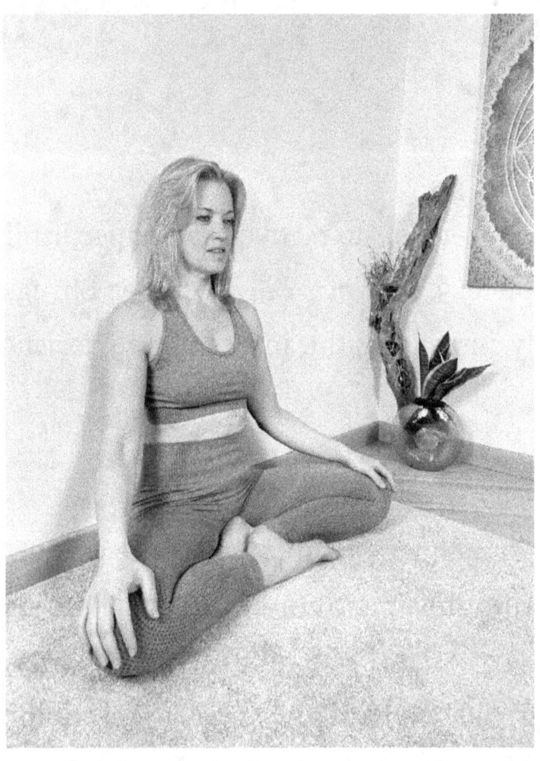 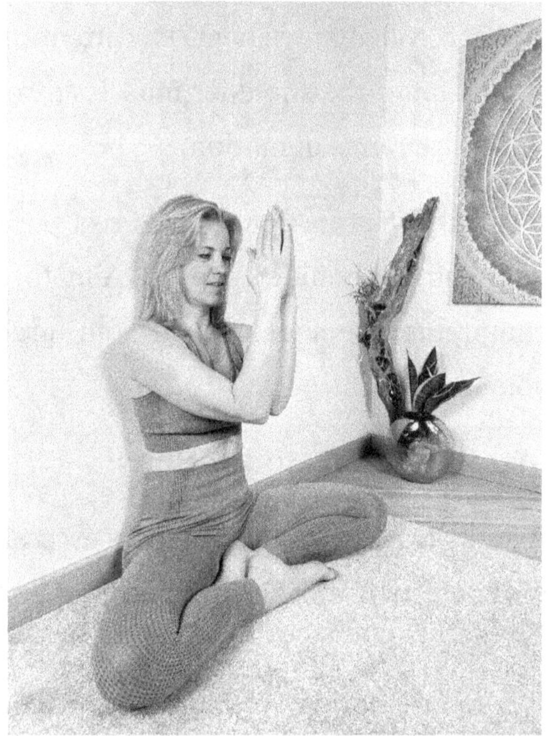

1. **Starting Position:** Sit on the floor with your legs crossed and your spine straight against the wall. This position ensures stability and support during the exercise.

2. **Arm Position:** Bring your arms up toward your chest, palms facing up and touching as if you were praying. Connect your elbows to maintain a compact and controlled starting position.

3. **Breathing:** Prioritize mindful breathing. Bring your focus to your breath, establishing a rhythm that complements the pulsating movement. Conscious breathing enhances the mind-body connection.

4. **Pulsating Movement:** Slowly and carefully lift your connected arms up toward the ceiling. Once at the peak, quickly return your arms to chest height. This rapid pulsing movement intensifies the engagement of your arm and shoulder muscles.

5. **Repeat:** Continue this lifting and pulsing motion for 10 repetitions initially, gradually working your way up to 20 repetitions. Maintain a steady and controlled pace to maximize the advantages of the exercise.

6. **Finishing Position:** After completing the desired number of repetitions, lower your arms back down to chest height, keeping the pulsating action controlled and deliberate.

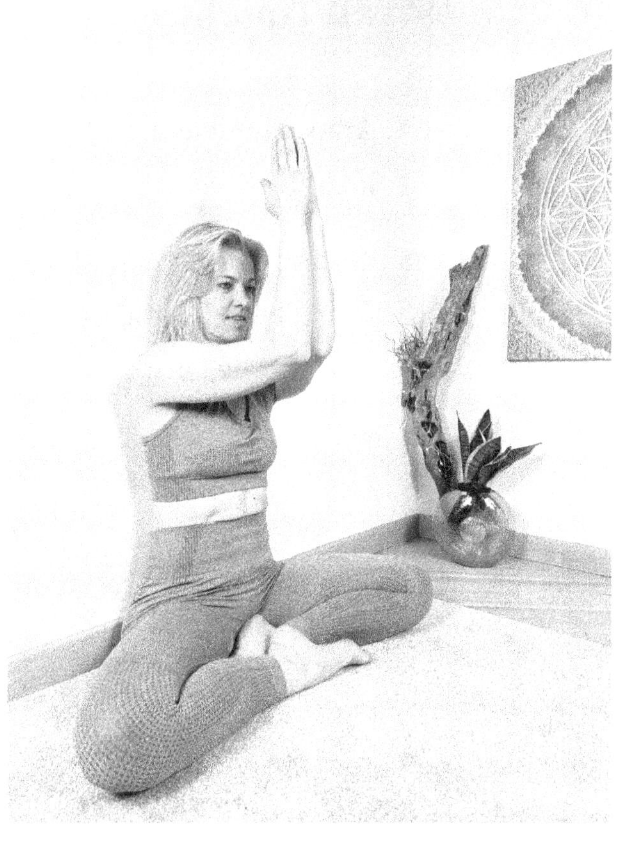

Warnings and Contraindications:

- Avoid straining your neck or shoulders during the Prayer Pulse exercise. Focus on using your arm muscles to lift and pulse, rather than pulling with your neck or shrugging your shoulders.
- Individuals with shoulder injuries or conditions, such as rotator cuff issues or impingement, should use caution when performing this exercise and may need to modify the range of motion or intensity to avoid exacerbating their condition.

Advanced Version:

- **Extended Range of Motion:** Instead of stopping at chest height, extend your arms fully overhead during the lifting phase. This increases the distance your muscles must travel, adding intensity and requiring greater strength and control.

36 Plank Wall Touches

Affected Area: Arms, Shoulders, and Core.

Objectives of the Exercise: Plank Wall Touches elevate the traditional plank exercise by adding a dynamic arm movement, focusing on sculpting the arms and shoulders while maintaining core strength. By incorporating the wall, this exercise provides stability and support, making it accessible for various fitness levels.

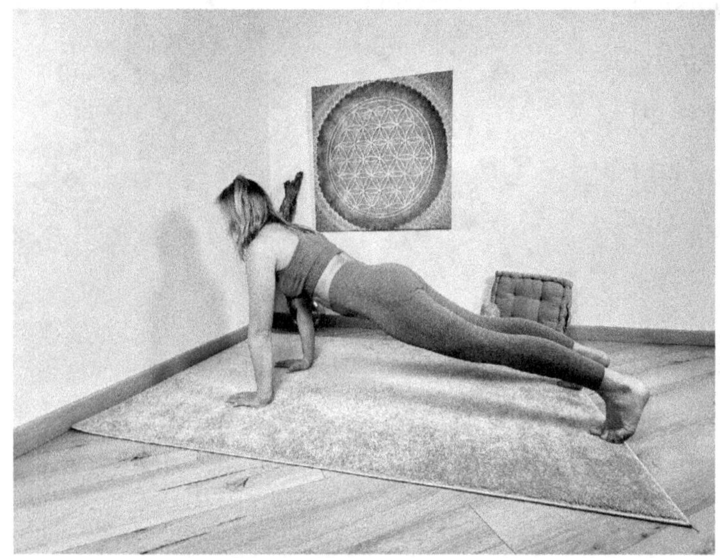

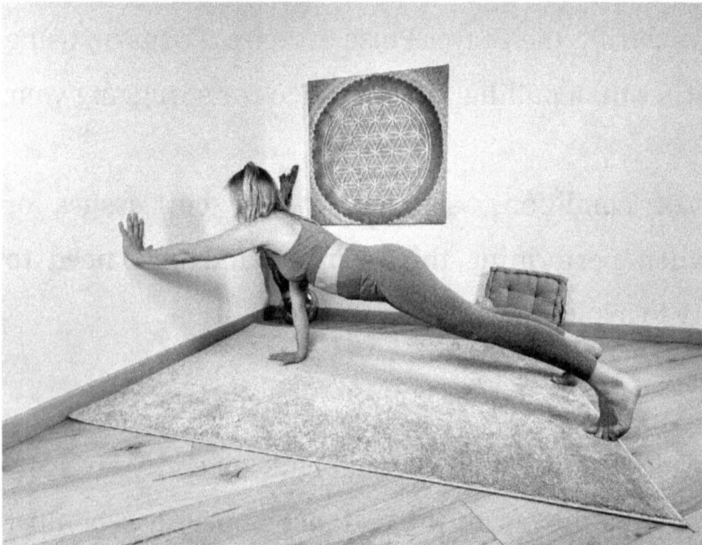

Step-by-Step Instructions:

1. **Starting Position:** Assume a plank position with your feet together and arms straight, positioned just below your shoulders. Your body should be approximately one arm's distance from the wall.

2. **Hand Movement:** Lift one hand from the floor and tap it on the wall in front of you. Maintain a straight trunk throughout this movement, ensuring your core remains engaged. This action requires controlled strength and balance.

3. **Return to Starting Position:** After tapping the wall, smoothly return the lifted hand to its initial position on the floor. Ensure a controlled and deliberate movement to maximize muscle engagement.

4. **Alternate Hands:** Repeat the process with the opposite hand. Lift and tap, then return to the starting plank position. Continue alternating between hands, creating a rhythmic pattern.

5. **Repetitions:** Perform the Plank Wall Touches for 15 repetitions, focusing on precision and controlled movements. This exercise is not about speed but rather the quality of each touch and return.

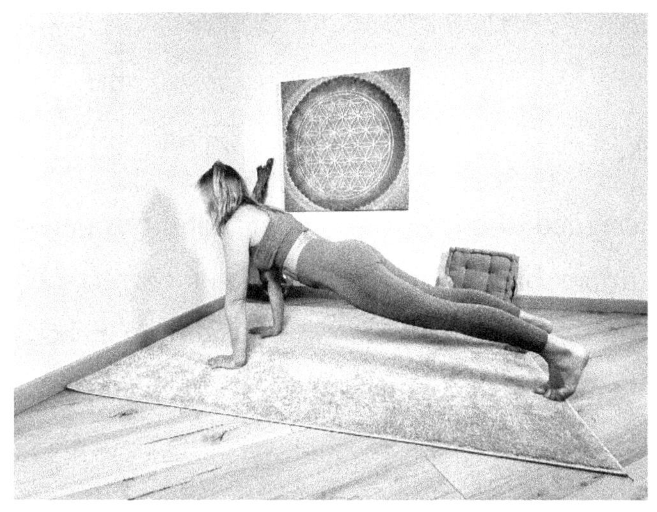 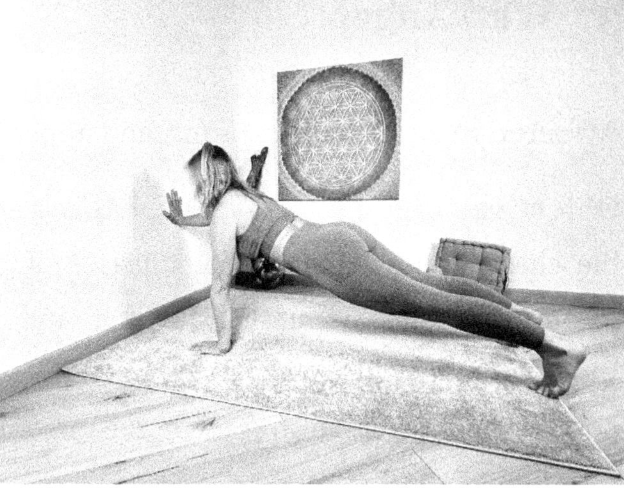

Warnings and Contraindications:

- Ensure that your wrists, elbows, and shoulders are properly aligned to prevent strain or injury.
- Avoid overarching or sagging your lower back during the movement. Maintain a straight line from head to heels to protect your spine.

Advanced Version:

- **Touch the wall with both hands:** after placing one hand on the wall, place the other hand as well and hold the position for a few seconds, then gently lower one hand and then the other. Repeat for 20 repetitions.

37 Wall Angels

Affected area: Shoulders, arms, and upper back.

Objectives of the Exercise: Wall Angels are designed to improve shoulder mobility, open up the chest, and strengthen the muscles of the upper back. This exercise helps correct poor posture, enhance shoulder stability, and promote better alignment of the upper body. Incorporating Wall Angels into your routine can lead to reduced shoulder tightness, improved posture, and increased strength in the upper back muscles.

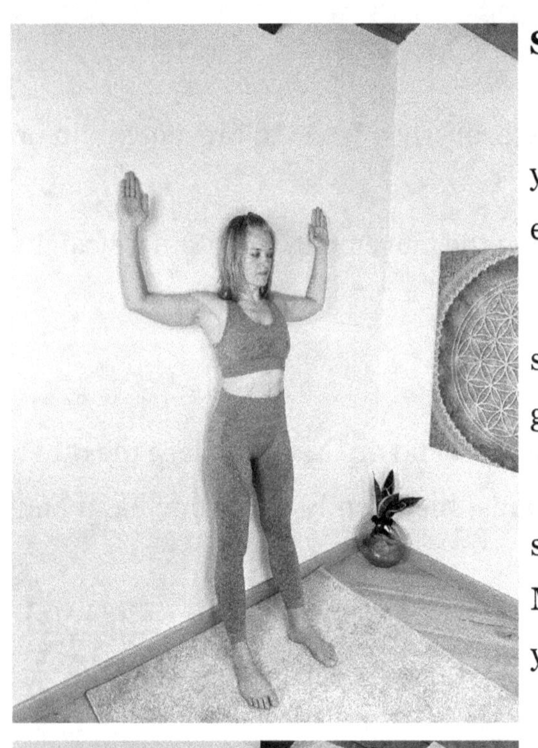

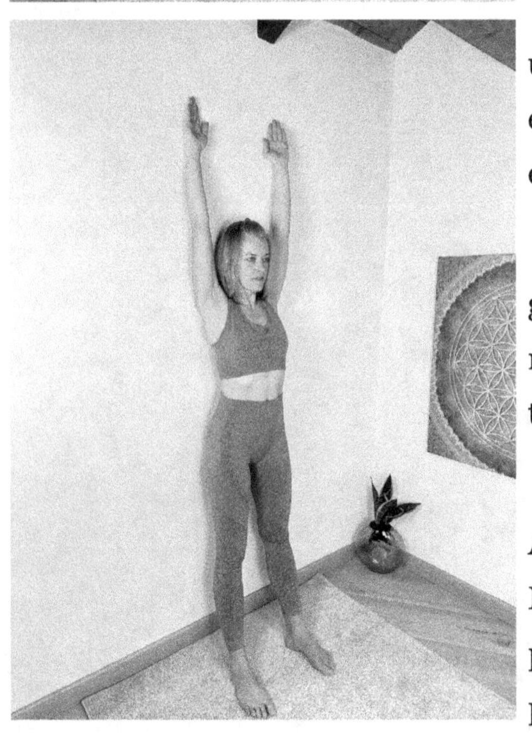

Step-by-Step Instructions:

1. **Starting Position:** Stand facing the wall, with your feet a few inches away and hip-width apart. Your entire back should be in contact with the wall.

2. **Arm Placement:** Extend your arms sideways at shoulder level, with palms facing forward and fingertips gently touching the wall.

3. **Upward Motion:** Initiate the movement by smoothly sliding your arms upward along the wall. Maintain contact with your elbows and wrists, ensuring your arms stay aligned with your shoulders.

4. **Full Extension:** Continue the upward motion until your range of motion allows, aiming for full arm extension without arching your lower back or losing contact with the wall.

5. **Downward Motion:** Reverse the motion by gently sliding your arms back down to shoulder height, maintaining contact with your elbows and wrists throughout the descent.

6. **Repetitions:** Complete 10-12 repetitions of Wall Angels, emphasizing controlled and deliberate motions. Move slowly and smoothly through each repetition, paying attention to your breathing and maintaining proper form.

Warnings and Contraindications:

- Avoid overarching your lower back or leaning forward excessively during Wall Angels. Remember to keep your spine in a neutral position and activate your core muscles to support your upper body throughout the exercise.
- Individuals with limited shoulder mobility or range of motion may need to modify the exercise by reducing the range of motion or performing the movement with lighter resistance. Listen to your body and adjust the exercise as needed to avoid straining the shoulder joints.

Advanced Version:

To advance the Wall Angels and increase the challenge, you can incorporate the following modifications:

- **Single-Arm Wall Angels:** Perform Wall Angels with one arm at a time while keeping the opposite arm stationary. This unilateral variation helps correct muscle imbalances and improves overall shoulder stability.

38 Long Arms Pulses

Affected area: Arms and shoulders.

Objectives of the Exercise: Long Arms Pulses is a targeted exercise designed to tone and strengthen the muscles in your arms and shoulders. The controlled pulsating movement, combined with the supportive stance against the wall, provides an effective workout for achieving sleek and defined upper arms. This exercise emphasizes both the chest and biceps, offering a comprehensive approach to upper body sculpting. By incorporating breath awareness and mindful pulsing, Long Arms Pulses not only shapes your physique but also enhances your mind-body connection.

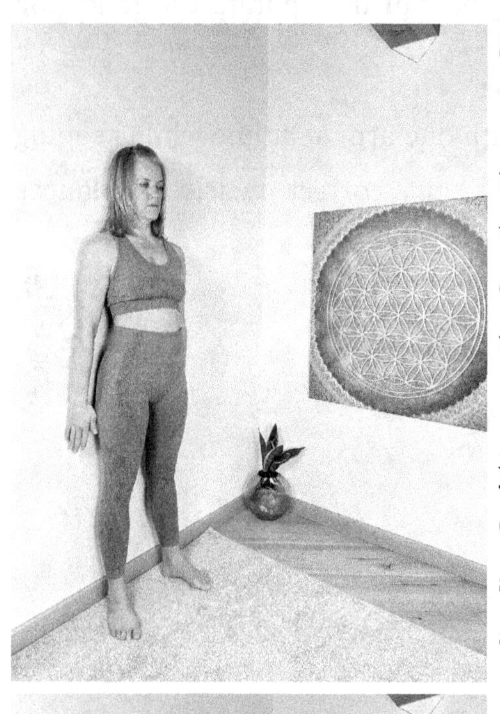

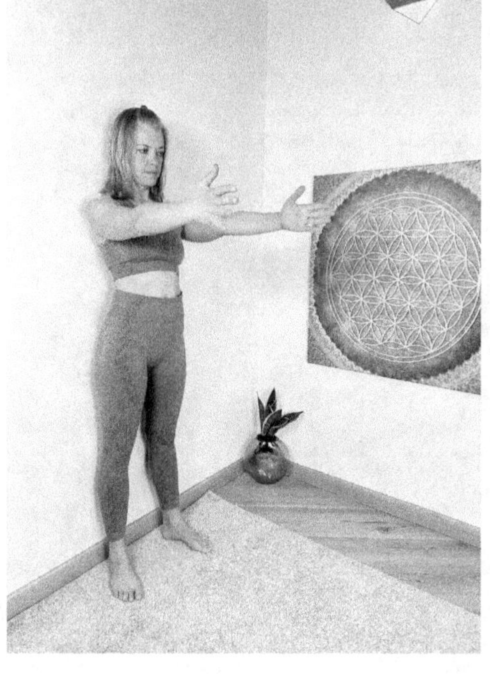

Step-by-Step Instructions:

1. **Starting Position:** Stand with your back against the wall, ensuring that your buttocks are in contact with the wall surface. Keep a slight bend in your knees and actively engage your core muscles to maintain stability throughout the duration of the exercise.

2. **Arm Position:** Slowly lift your arms out in front of you, keeping them straight with palms facing inward. Continue the upward motion until your arms are at shoulder height and directly in front of your chest. Your arms should be parallel to the floor.

3. **Breathing:** At the peak of the arm elevation, take a deep breath in. This inhalation prepares your body for the pulsating movement.

4. **Pulsating Movement:** As you breathe out, initiate a slow pulsating movement by bringing your arms slightly inward. Focus on engaging the muscles in your chest and biceps during this controlled pulsing action. Imagine squeezing your chest and biceps as you bring your arms closer together.

5. **Pulsing Count:** Pulse your arms for 10 counts, maintaining precision and control. The pulsing movement

should be deliberate, emphasizing the contraction of the targeted muscles. Ensure that your shoulders remain relaxed and your elbows slightly bent throughout the pulsing motion.

6. **Rest Period:** After completing the pulsing sequence, rest for 10 counts while maintaining your arms at shoulder height. Use this rest period to catch your breath and prepare for the next repetition.

7. **Repetitions:** Repeat the entire process for a total of 3 full 10 count repetitions. Focus on maintaining proper form and controlled breathing throughout each repetition.

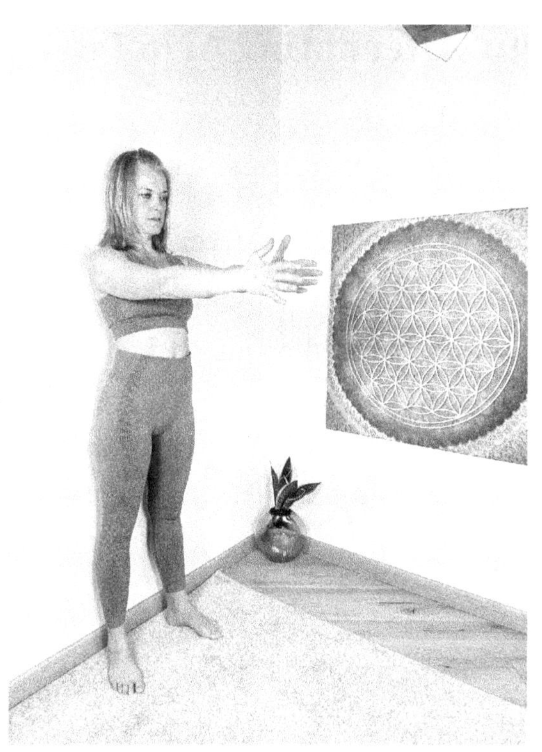

Warnings and Contraindications:

- If you have any shoulder or arm injuries, exercise caution when performing Long Arms Pulses. Commence with lighter weights or resistance, progressively advancing as you develop strength and confidence. Avoid any movements that cause pain or discomfort in the shoulder joints.
- Refrain from locking your elbows or hyperextending your arms during the exercise. Maintain a slight bend in your elbows to reduce joint strain and prevent potential injuries.

Advanced Version:

- **Extended Duration:** Increase the duration of each pulsing sequence from 10 counts to 15 or 20 counts. The longer pulsing duration will challenge your muscles to work harder and improve endurance.

39 Alternating Arm Push-Ups

Affected area: Arms, shoulders, and chest.

Objectives of the Exercise: Alternating Arm Push-Ups against the wall focus on building strength in the shoulders, arms, and chest. This dynamic exercise incorporates unilateral movements, adding an extra challenge to standard push-ups. By alternating arms, it promotes balanced muscle development and enhances overall upper body strength.

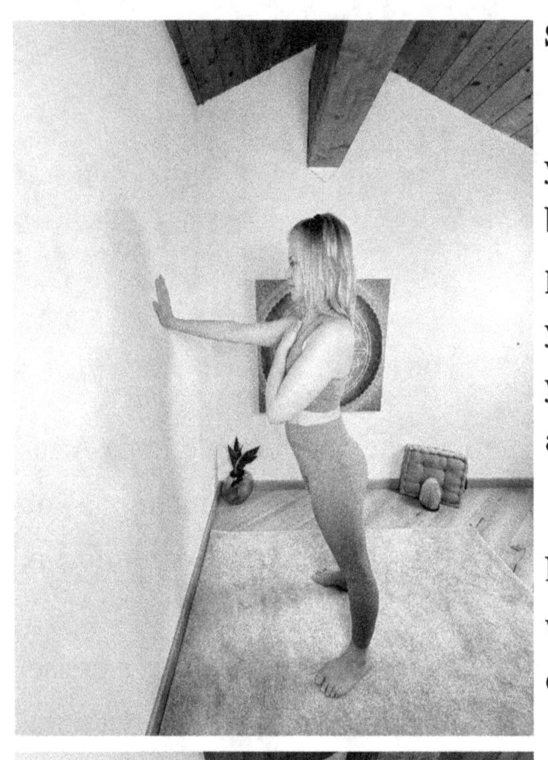

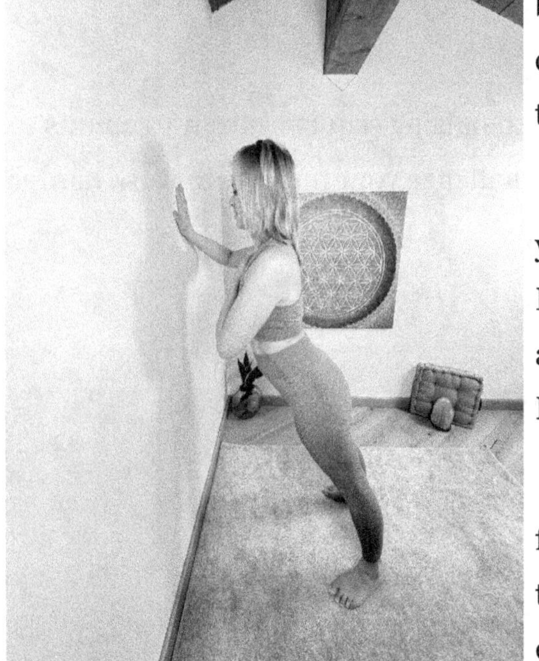

Step-by-Step Instructions:

1. **Starting Position:** Face the wall and position yourself around an arm's length away from it. After bringing your arms up to shoulder height, press your palms on the wall at a distance equal to the width of your shoulders. A straight line should be formed from your head to your heels, and your feet should be spaced at a distance equal to the breadth of your hips.

2. **Hand Placement:** Begin by placing your left hand on your right shoulder, and your right hand on the wall in front of you. Keep your left elbow pointed outward, parallel to the floor.

3. **Breathing:** Breathe in deeply, preparing your body for the movement. Upon exhaling, engage your core muscles and maintain a steady breath throughout the exercise.

4. **Movement - Right Arm:** Exhale as you lower your chest toward the wall by bending your right elbow. Keep your body in a straight line from head to heels, avoiding any arching or sagging in the lower back. Lower yourself until your chest gently touches the wall.

5. **Hold and Contract:** Hold the lowered position for two counts, focusing on engaging your chest and triceps. Feel the muscles working as you maintain control and stability.

6. **Movement - Right Arm:** Breathe in as you push yourself back to the starting position by straightening your right arm. Keep your movements smooth and controlled, using the strength of your chest and triceps to return to the starting position.

7. **Hand Placement - Left Arm:** Now, switch the position of your arms. Put your right hand on your left shoulder, and your left hand on the wall in front of you. Ensure that your left hand is at shoulder height and shoulder-width apart.

8. **Movement - Left Arm:** Exhale as you lower your chest toward the wall by bending your left elbow. Maintain a straight line from head to heels and focus on the contraction in your chest and triceps as you lower yourself.

9. **Hold and Contract:** Hold the lowered position for two counts, continuing to engage your muscles. Keep your core tight and your body stable throughout the movement.

10. **Repeat Alternating Motion:** Continue this alternating motion, swapping arms for each repetition. Aim to perform 10 repetitions on each arm, totaling 20 alternating arm push-ups.

Warnings and Contraindications:

- If you have shoulder, arm, or wrist injuries, exercise caution while engaging in Alternating Arm Push-Ups. Begin with a limited range.
- Ensure you avoid overextending or allowing your lower back to sag during the movement. Keep your core activated and maintain proper spinal alignment to minimize the risk of strain or injury.

Advanced Version:

- **Increase Repetitions:** Gradually increase the number of repetitions on each arm, aiming for 12-15 repetitions per arm. This increases the overall workload and endurance of the muscles involved.

40 Open Arm Wall Pulses

Affected Area: Arms and Shoulders.

Objectives of the Exercise: Open Arm Wall Pulses are designed to target the muscles in the arms and shoulders, promoting strength, definition, and improved mobility. By utilizing the support of the wall, this exercise provides stability while isolating specific muscle groups for effective toning and sculpting.

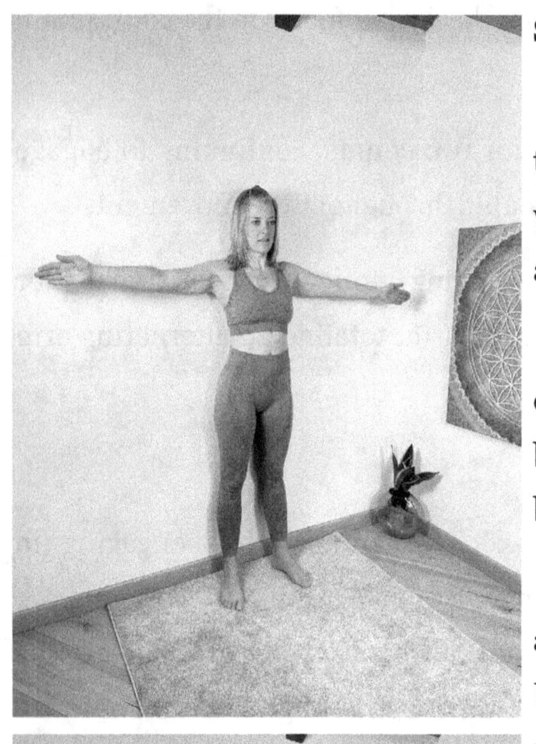

Step-by-Step Instructions:

1. **Starting Position:** Stand with your back against the wall, ensuring your glutes are in contact with the wall. Maintain stability throughout the exercise by actively engaging your core muscles.

2. **Arm Positioning:** Slide your arms up the wall on either side of you, keeping your elbows locked and the backs of your hands against the wall. Your arms should be extended straight, parallel to the floor.

3. **Rotational Movement:** Rotate your palms from a palms-outward position to a palms-upward position. Use your shoulder and arm muscles to initiate this rotational movement. Ensure that your shoulder blades remain in contact with the wall throughout the exercise.

4. **Pulsing Movement:** Perform the pulsing movement for 10 counts, focusing on controlled and precise rotations. Emphasize engagement in the shoulder and arm muscles during each repetition.

5. **Rest and Repeat:** After completing the pulsing sequence, rest for 10 counts while maintaining proper posture and core engagement. Repeat the entire process for a total of 3 full 10-count repetitions.

Warnings and Contraindications:

- Steer clear of overextending or allowing your lower back to sag during the movement. Ensure your core remains engaged, and maintain proper spinal alignment to minimize the risk of strain or injury.

Advanced Version:

- **Increased Range of Motion:** Extend the range of motion by moving your arms in a larger arc during the pulsing movement. Begin with palms facing outward, then rotate backward until your palms are facing upward. This extended range intensifies the engagement of your shoulder and arm muscles, enhancing both strength and flexibility.

Chapter 3

28-Day Workout (Beginners)

Welcome to the 28-Day Beginner Workout Challenge, where we'll be incorporating Pilates exercises with the support of a wall to kickstart your fitness journey! Before we dive in, it's crucial to begin with a short warm-up to prepare your body for the upcoming challenge.

Start by gently marching in place or taking a brisk walk for 5-10 minutes to increase your heart rate and warm up your muscles. Follow this with some dynamic stretches, such as those discussed earlier, to further loosen up your body.

As you embark on this 28-day adventure, remember to listen to your body and honor your limits. Stay consistent, but don't be afraid to modify exercises or take breaks as needed. Progression comes with time, so focus on gradual improvement rather than pushing yourself too hard too soon.

Embrace the journey ahead with enthusiasm and determination. Each day presents an opportunity to grow stronger and more confident in your abilities. With dedication and perseverance, you'll soon discover the transformative power of Pilates and the support of the wall in achieving your fitness goals.

Day 1:

Exercise	Reference Page	Repetitions
Wall Roll Downs	26	8
Wall Plank	46	20 sec
Wall Squats	66	10
Wall Push-Ups	90	8
Wall Shoulder Shrugs	92	10

Day 2:

Exercise	Reference Page	Repetitions
Wall Pike	28	8
Wall Side Plank	48	20 sec
Split Squats	68	10 (each leg)
Prayer Pulse	94	10
Plank Wall Touches	96	10

Day 3:

Exercise	Reference Page	Repetitions
Wall Walk	30	5 steps
Wall Crunches	50	12
Wall Sit with Alternating Leg Extension	70	10 (each leg)
Wall 100s	52	10 (cycles)
Wall Angels	98	10

Day 4:

Exercise	Reference Page	Repetitions
Triceps Push-Up With Side Leg Lift	32	8 (each side)
Toe Touches	54	12
Wall Sit Calf Raises	72	15
Wall Shoulder Shrugs	92	10
Alternating Arm Push-Ups	102	8 (each arm)

Day 5:

Exercise	Reference Page	Repetitions
Wall Sit with Arm Raises	34	10
Wall Bicycle	56	12
Wall Single-Leg Lifts	74	8 (each leg)
Long Arms Pulses	100	15

| Open Arm Wall Pulses | 104 | 12 |

Day 6:

Exercise	Reference Page	Repetitions
Roll-Up into Bridge	36	8
Wall Twist	60	10
Wall-Supported Dynamic Back Lunge	76	10 (each leg)
Prayer Pulse	94	10
Plank Wall Touches	96	10

Day 7: REST AND RECOVERY

Day 8:

Exercise	Reference Page	Repetitions
Single-Leg Bridge with Abduction	38	8 (each leg)
Wall Sit Calf Raises	72	15
Wall-Supported Side Kicks	78	10 (each leg)
Wall Push-Ups	90	8
Wall Angels	98	10

Day 9:

Exercise	Reference Page	Repetitions
Kneeling Side Leg Lift	40	10 (each leg)
Side Plank with Rotation	42	20 sec (each side)
Wall Lateral Squat	80	10 (each leg)
Wall Shoulder Shrugs	92	10
Alternating Arm Push-Ups	102	8 (each arm)

Day 10:

Exercise	Reference Page	Repetitions
Wall Plank	46	20 sec
Quadruped Leg Extension	88	10 (each leg)
Wall Sit with Alternating Leg Extension	70	12
Prayer Pulse	94	10
Wall Sit Calf Raises	72	15

Day 11:

Exercise	Reference Page	Repetitions
Wall 100s	52	10
Wall Crunches	50	15
Wall Single-Leg Lifts	74	10 (each leg)
Leg Slides	86	12
Wall Bridge	84	8

Day 12:

Exercise	Reference Page	Repetitions
Wall Pike	28	10
Wall Squats	66	15
Wall Push-Ups	90	12
Wall Lateral Squat	80	12 (each leg)
Lying Windshield Wipers	58	12

Day 13:

Exercise	Reference Page	Repetitions
Wall Walk	30	8
Wall Twist	60	10
Standing Knee Raises	64	20
Alternating Arm Push-Ups	102	10 (each arm)

Wall-Supported Dynamic Back Lunge	76	10 (each leg)

Day 14: REST AND RECOVERY

Day 15:

Exercise	Reference Page	Repetitions
Roll-Up into Bridge	36	10
Wall Bicycle	56	12
Prayer Pulse	94	10
Wall 100s	52	10
Wall Sit Calf Raises	72	15
Wall Plank	46	20 sec
Wall Crunches	50	15

Day 16:

Exercise	Reference Page	Repetitions
Wall-Supported Side Kicks	78	12 (each leg)
Wall Sit with Arm Raises	34	12
Wall Shoulder Shrugs	92	12
Plank Wall Touches	96	10 (each arm)
Wall Twist	60	10
Wall Pike	28	10
Wall Sit with Alternating Leg Extension	70	12

Day 17:

Exercise	Reference Page	Repetitions
Wall Angels	98	12
Alternating Arm Push-Ups	102	10 (each arm)
Wall Single-Leg Lifts	74	10 (each leg)
Wall-Supported Dynamic Back Lunge	76	10 (each leg)
Wall Squats	66	15

| Wall Roll Downs | 26 | 10 |
| Wall Lateral Squat | 80 | 12 (each leg) |

Day 18:

Exercise	Reference Page	Repetitions
Reach Backs	44	10
Quadruped Leg Extension	88	10 (each leg)
Wall Sit Calf Raises	72	15
Wall Plank	46	20 sec
Wall Crunches	50	15
Wall Bridge	84	8
Roll-Up into Bridge	36	10

Day 19:

Exercise	Reference Page	Repetitions
Toe Touches	54	12
Wall Bicycle	56	12
Prayer Pulse	94	10
Wall 100s	52	10
Lying Windshield Wipers	58	12
Kneeling Side Leg Lift	40	10 (each leg)
Leg Slides	86	12

Day 20:

Exercise	Reference Page	Repetitions
Wall-Supported Side Kicks	78	12 (each leg)
Wall Sit with Arm Raises	72	12
Wall Shoulder Shrugs	92	12
Plank Wall Touches	96	10 (each arm)
Wall Twist	60	10

	28	10
Wall Pike	28	10
Wall Sit with Alternating Leg Extension	70	12

Day 21: REST AND RECOVERY

Day 22:

Exercise	Reference Page	Repetitions
Wall Angels	98	12
Alternating Arm Push-Ups	102	10 (each arm)
Wall Single-Leg Lifts	74	10 (each leg)
Wall-Supported Dynamic Back Lunge	76	10 (each leg)
Wall Squats	66	15
Single-Leg Bridge with Abduction	38	8 (each leg)
Wall Lateral Squat	80	12 (each leg)

Day 23:

Exercise	Reference Page	Repetitions
Reach Backs	44	10
Prayer Pulse	94	10
Wall Sit Calf Raises	72	15
Plank Wall Touches	96	10
Wall Crunches	50	15
Wall Bridge	84	8
Roll-Up into Bridge	36	10

Day 24:

Exercise	Reference Page	Repetitions
Standing Knee Raises	64	20
Wall Walk	30	10 steps
Quadruped Leg Extension	88	10 (each leg)
Lying Windshield Wipers	58	12

Split Squats	68	10 (each side)
Wall Twist	60	12
Wall Bicycle	56	12

Day 25:

Exercise	Reference Page	Repetitions
Wall Push-Ups	90	12
Wall Side Plank	48	20 sec (each side)
Wall Roll Downs	26	10
Wall-Supported Dynamic Back Lunge	76	10 (each leg)
Toe Touches	54	12
Wall Sit Calf Raises	72	15
Wall Pike	28	12

Day 26:

Exercise	Reference Page	Repetitions
Wall Crunches	50	12
Wall Lateral Squat	80	12
Wall 100s	52	15
Wall Angels	98	12
Wall Shoulder Shrugs	92	12
Marching Bridge	62	12
Wall-Supported Side Kicks	78	10 (each side)

Day 27:

Exercise	Reference Page	Repetitions
Wall Single-Leg Lifts	74	10 (each side)
Alternating Arm Push-Ups	102	10 (each side)
Single-Leg Bridge with Abduction	38	8 (each leg)
Leg Slides	86	12

Long Arms Pulses	100	12
Wall Sit with Arm Raises	34	12
Plank Wall Touches	96	12

Day 28: Dedicate this day to reflection, mindfulness, and gratitude. Take a few moments to contemplate the progress you've achieved, both physically and mentally, throughout the 28-day challenge. Reflect on any shifts in your mindset, energy levels, and overall well-being.

Chapter 4:

7-Day Workout (Advanced Level)

Welcome to the 7-Day Advanced Level Workout! This program is designed to challenge your strength, endurance, and flexibility with advanced Pilates exercises utilizing the support of a wall. Get ready to push your limits and take your fitness to new heights. Each day, you'll engage in targeted workouts tailored to sculpt and tone your body while enhancing overall performance. With dedication and determination, you'll conquer each session and emerge stronger than ever.

Day 1:

Exercise	Reference Page	Repetitions
Wall Pike	28	25
Wall Side Plank	48	35 sec (each side)
Wall Bridge	84	30
Wall Sit Calf Raises	72	30
Wall-Supported Dynamic Back Lunge	76	20 (each leg)
Wall Angels	98	25
Open Arm Wall Pulses	104	25
Long Arms Pulses	100	25
Plank Wall Touches	96	22
Alternating Arm Push-Ups	102	20

Day 2

Exercise	Reference Page	Repetitions
Wall Walk	30	15 steps
Roll-Up into Bridge	36	20
Wall Sit with Arm Raises	34	25
Wall Pike	28	20

Wall 100s	52	25
Wall Twist	60	22
Wall Bicycle	56	25
Prayer Pulse	94	20
Standing Knee Raises	64	30
Wall Bridge	84	25

Day 3

Exercise	Reference Page	Repetitions
Wall Roll Downs	26	22
Single-Leg Bridge with Abduction	38	20 (each side)
Side Plank with Rotation	42	30 sec (each side)
Reach Backs	44	22
Wall Crunches	50	30
Toe Touches	54	30
Wall Lateral Squat	80	30
Sumo Squat Pulses	82	30
Wall Push-Ups	90	25
Wall Sit with Alternating Leg Extension	70	18 (each side)

Day 4: REST AND RECOVERY

Day 5:

Exercise	Reference Page	Repetitions
Wall Roll Downs	26	20
Wall Squats	66	22
Wall Sit with Alternating Leg Extension	70	15 (each side)
Wall Sit Calf Raises	72	25
Wall-Supported Dynamic Back Lunge	76	20 (each leg)
Wall Lateral Squat	80	25
Sumo Squat Pulses	82	25

Wall Bridge	84	25
Long Arms Pulses	100	22
Plank Wall Touches	96	20

Day 6:

Exercise	Reference Page	Repetitions
Wall Plank	46	30 sec (each side)
Wall Crunches	50	25
Toe Touches	54	25
Lying Windshield Wipers	58	20
Marching Bridge	62	18 (each side)
Standing Knee Raises	64	30
Wall Push-Ups	90	18
Wall Shoulder Shrugs	92	20
Wall Angels	98	20
Open Arm Wall Pulses	104	20

Day 7:

Exercise	Reference Page	Repetitions
Wall Pike	28	18
Wall Walk	30	12 steps
Single-Leg Bridge with Abduction	38	15 (each side)
Side Plank with Rotation	42	25 sec (each side)
Reach Backs	44	18
Wall 100s	52	20
Wall Bicycle	56	22
Wall Twist	60	20
Roll-Up into Bridge	36	18
Triceps Push-Up With Side Leg Lift	32	15 (each side)

Chapter 5

BONUS WORKOUT: 7-Day Abdominal Core (Beginner And Advanced)

Get ready to sculpt and strengthen your core with this bonus 7-Day Abdominal Core Workout! This program is specially crafted to strengthen your core abdominals and back muscles, promoting stability and overall strength. With a focus on targeted exercises, you'll engage in movements designed to tone and sculpt your midsection while improving posture and reducing the risk of injury.

BEGINNER

Day 1:

Exercise	Reference Page	Repetitions
Wall Plank	46	30 sec
Wall Crunches	50	15
Toe Touches	54	15
Wall 100s	52	10
Wall Twist	60	15 (each side)

Day 2:

Exercise	Reference Page	Repetitions
Wall Side Plank	48	20 sec (each side)
Wall Bicycle	56	12 (each side)
Lying Windshield Wipers	58	10 (each side)
Standing Knee Raises	64	30
Wall Roll Downs	26	10

Day 3:

Exercise	Reference Page	Repetitions
Wall Sit with Arm Raises	34	15
Wall Walk	30	5 steps
Reach Backs	44	10
Marching Bridge	62	12 (each side)
Roll-Up into Bridge	36	8

Day 4: REST AND RECOVERY

Day 5:

Exercise	Reference Page	Repetitions
Wall Plank	46	30 sec
Wall Bicycle	56	15 (each side)
Wall Crunches	50	15
Marching Bridge	62	12 (each side)
Side Plank with Rotation	42	20 sec (each side)
Standing Knee Raises	64	30
Wall Roll Downs	26	10

Day 6:

Exercise	Reference Page	Repetitions
Wall Sit with Arm Raises	34	15
Toe Touches	54	20
Single-Leg Bridge with Abduction	38	10 (each side)
Wall 100s	52	15
Wall Pike	28	10
Wall Twist	60	15 (each side)
Kneeling Side Leg Lift	40	12 (each side)

Day 7:

Exercise	Reference Page	Repetitions
Wall Side Plank	48	25 sec (each side)
Reach Backs	44	12
Wall Walk	30	8 steps
Lying Windshield Wipers	58	12 (each side)
Roll-Up into Bridge	36	10
Triceps Push-Up With Side Leg Lift	32	8 (each side)
Wall Crunches	50	20

ADVANCED

Day 1:

Exercise	Reference Page	Repetitions
Wall Pike	28	15
Wall 100s	52	20
Wall Twist	60	20 (each side)
Wall Crunches	50	20
Wall Bicycle	56	25 (each side)
Wall Side Plank	48	30 sec (each side)
Wall Roll Downs	26	12
Reach Backs	44	15

Day 2:

Exercise	Reference Page	Repetitions
Roll-Up into Bridge	36	15
Marching Bridge	62	15 (each side)
Wall Walk	30	10 steps
Side Plank with Rotation	42	30 sec (each side)
Standing Knee Raises	64	25
Toe Touches	54	25
Single-Leg Bridge with Abduction	38	12 (each side)
Triceps Push-Up With Side Leg Lift	32	12 (each side)

Day 3:

Exercise	Reference Page	Repetitions
Wall Plank	46	40 sec
Kneeling Side Leg Lift	40	15 (each side)
Lying Windshield Wipers	58	20 (each side)
Wall Sit with Arm Raises	34	20
Wall Twist	60	25 (each side)
Single-Leg Bridge with Abduction	38	15 (each side)
Wall Pike	28	15

Day 4: REST AND RECOVERY

Day 5:

Exercise	Reference Page	Repetitions
Wall Pike	28	18
Wall 100s	52	25
Wall Twist	60	25 (each side)
Wall Crunches	50	25
Wall Bicycle	56	30 (each side)
Wall Side Plank	48	45 sec (each side)

Wall Roll Downs	26	15
Reach Backs	44	18
Wall Walk	30	12 steps
Roll-Up into Bridge	36	18

Day 6:

Exercise	Reference Page	Repetitions
Side Plank with Rotation	42	45 sec (each side)
Standing Knee Raises	64	25
Toe Touches	54	30
Wall Plank	46	50 sec
Wall Sit with Arm Raises	34	25
Wall Pike	28	20
Lying Windshield Wipers	58	25 (each side)
Wall Bicycle	56	35 (each side)
Single-Leg Bridge with Abduction	38	15 (each side)
Triceps Push-Up With Side Leg Lift	32	15 (each side)

Day 7:

Exercise	Reference Page	Repetitions
Wall Crunches	50	30
Wall Twist	60	30 (each side)
Wall 100s	52	30
Marching Bridge	62	20 (each side)
Wall Side Plank	48	60 sec (each side)
Wall Roll Downs	26	20
Wall Walk	30	15 steps
Wall Pike	28	22
Reach Backs	44	20
Wall Sit with Arm Raises	34	30

Chapter 6:

BONUS: Nutritional Tips

Welcome to the bonus chapter on nutritional tips—a crucial component of your journey to optimal health, vitality, and success in Wall Pilates. While exercise plays a vital role in achieving your fitness goals, it's essential to recognize that nutrition is equally important, if not more so, in supporting your overall well-being and maximizing your performance. In this chapter, we'll delve into the symbiotic relationship between exercise and nutrition, explore the key principles of a healthy diet, and provide practical tips and strategies to fuel your body for success in your Wall Pilates practice.

The Link Between Nutrition and Exercise

Before we dive into the specifics of nutrition, let's take a moment to understand the connection between diet and exercise. While exercise provides the stimulus for physical change and improvement, it's nutrition that provides the raw materials your body needs to repair, recover, and adapt to the demands of training. Without adequate nutrition, your body may struggle to perform optimally, hindering your progress and potentially leading to fatigue, injury, or burnout.

The Importance of a Balanced Diet

Achieving optimal health and performance hinges on maintaining a balanced diet, which supplies your body with essential nutrients for flourishing. Strive to consume a diverse array of nutrient-rich foods from every food group into your meals, encompassing fruits, vegetables, lean proteins, whole grains, and healthy fats. Prioritize whole, minimally processed foods, and limit your intake of refined sugars, saturated fats, and processed foods, which offer little nutritional value and can negatively impact your health and well-being.

Key Nutritional Principles for Wall Pilates

As you begin your Wall Pilates journey, consider the following nutritional principles to bolster your success and optimize your performance:

> **Hydration is Key:** Proper hydration is essential for optimal performance and recovery in Wall Pilates. Make an effort to stay well-hydrated by drinking ample water

throughout the day, especially before, during, and after your workouts. This helps maintain hydration levels and replaces fluids lost through perspiration.

Balance Your Macronutrients: Your body requires a balance of carbohydrates, proteins, and fats to fuel your workouts, support muscle repair and growth, and maintain overall health. Aim to include a source of each macronutrient in every meal or snack to ensure balanced energy levels and sustained performance.

Prioritize Protein: Protein is vital for muscle repair and growth, making it essential for anyone engaging in regular exercise, including Wall Pilates. To support muscle recovery and improve overall results, include lean protein sources like chicken, tofu, fish, beans, and lentils in your meals.

Fuel Your Workouts: Eating a small meal or snack containing carbohydrates and protein before your Wall Pilates workouts can help fuel your performance and enhance your endurance. Experiment with options such as a banana with nut butter, Greek yogurt with fruit, or a small turkey sandwich on whole-grain bread to find what works best for you.

Recover with Proper Nutrition: After your workouts, prioritize post-exercise nutrition to support muscle recovery and replenish glycogen stores. Aim to consume a combination of carbohydrates and protein within 30 minutes to an hour after your workout to maximize recovery and optimize your results.

Listen to Your Body: Pay attention to your body's hunger and satiety cues, and eat mindfully to fuel your body's needs. Avoid restrictive diets or overly rigid eating patterns, and instead focus on nourishing your body with wholesome, nutrient-rich foods that support your health and well-being.

Practical Nutritional Tips for Success

In addition to these key principles, here are some practical tips and strategies to help you fuel your body for success in your Wall Pilates practice:

Plan Ahead: Take the time to plan and prepare your meals and snacks in advance to ensure you have nutritious options readily available when hunger strikes. Batch cook meals, portion out snacks, and stock your pantry with healthy staples to make eating well easy and convenient.

Eat Mindfully: Practice mindful eating by tuning into your body's hunger and satiety signals, eating slowly, and savoring each bite. Avoid distractions such as screens or multitasking while eating, and focus on enjoying your meals and the nourishment they provide.

Stay Consistent: Consistency is key when it comes to nutrition, just as it is in your Wall Pilates practice. You should make it a goal to have regular, well-balanced meals and snacks throughout the day in order to keep your energy levels steady, to assist the healing of your muscles, and to maximize your performance.

Stay Hydrated: Hydration is essential for optimal performance and recovery in Wall Pilates. Keep a reusable water bottle with you throughout the day and aim to drink water regularly to stay hydrated and replenish fluids lost through sweat.

Listen to Your Body: Finally, listen to your body's signals and adjust your nutrition as needed to support your health and well-being. If you're feeling fatigued or sluggish, evaluate your diet and make adjustments to ensure you're meeting your body's needs for energy, nutrients, and hydration.

Sample Nutritional Plan

To help you get started, here's a sample nutritional plan to accompany your Wall Pilates workouts on various days:

Note: This is just a sample plan and should be customized based on your individual needs, preferences, and dietary requirements.

Breakfast:

- Option 1: Greek yogurt topped with berries and a sprinkle of nuts or seeds.
- Option 2: Whole grain toast with avocado and poached eggs.
- Option 3: Smoothie made with spinach, banana, almond milk, and protein powder.

Morning Snack:

- Option 1: Apple slices with almond butter.
- Option 2: Carrot sticks with hummus.
- Option 3: Handful of mixed nuts and seeds.

Lunch:

- Option 1: Quinoa salad with mixed vegetables, grilled chicken, and a drizzle of olive oil.
- Option 2: Whole grain wrap filled with turkey, lettuce, tomato, avocado, and mustard.
- Option 3: Lentil soup with whole grain crackers and a side salad.

Afternoon Snack:

- Option 1: Cottage cheese with pineapple chunks.
- Option 2: Rice cakes with mashed avocado and cherry tomatoes.
- Option 3: Greek yogurt with granola and sliced banana.

Dinner:

- Option 1: Baked salmon with roasted sweet potatoes and steamed broccoli.
- Option 2: Stir-fried tofu with mixed vegetables and brown rice.
- Option 3: Grilled chicken breast with quinoa pilaf and sautéed spinach.

Evening Snack (Optional):

- Option 1: Handful of cherry tomatoes with mozzarella cheese.
- Option 2: Sliced cucumber with hummus.
- Option 3: Air-popped popcorn sprinkled with nutritional yeast.

As you can see, nutrition plays a pivotal role in supporting your success and maximizing your performance in Wall Pilates. By fueling your body with nutritious, balanced meals and snacks, you can optimize your energy levels, support muscle recovery, and achieve your fitness goals with confidence and vitality. So, embrace the power of nutrition, prioritize nourishing your body with wholesome foods, and let your healthy eating habits fuel your journey to strength, resilience, and transformation in your Wall Pilates practice and beyond.

Chapter 7:

BONUS: 7 Breathing Exercises

In this chapter, we'll explore the profound impact of conscious breathing on both your Pilates practice and everyday life, and we'll introduce seven empowering breathing exercises to integrate seamlessly into your routine. So, let's harness the power of breath and elevate your practice to new heights!

The Importance of Conscious Breathing

In the context of Wall Pilates, conscious breathing serves as a powerful tool to enhance your practice, improve your focus and concentration, and deepen your mind-body connection. Beyond the mat, conscious breathing can also help you manage stress, regulate emotions, and cultivate a sense of calm and clarity in the face of life's challenges. By integrating breathing exercises into your Wall Pilates practice, you can unlock the full potential of your body and mind and experience profound transformation both on and off the mat.

Benefits of Conscious Breathing

The advantages of conscious breathing extend far beyond the physical realm—they encompass the entire spectrum of human experience, from the physical to the emotional, mental, and spiritual dimensions. By practicing conscious breathing, you can:

- **Improve Physical Performance:** Conscious breathing helps optimize oxygen delivery to your muscles, enhancing endurance, stamina, and performance during your Wall Pilates workouts.
- **Enhance Mind-Body Connection:** Conscious breathing fosters a deeper awareness of your body and its movements, allowing you to move with greater precision, control, and fluidity on the mat.
- **Reduce Stress and Anxiety:** Conscious breathing activates the body's relaxation response, promoting feelings of calm, relaxation, and emotional balance in stressful situations.
- **Increase Energy and Vitality:** Conscious breathing replenishes your body's energy stores, revitalizing your mind and body and increasing your overall sense of vitality and well-being.

- **Improve Focus and Concentration:** Conscious breathing enhances mental clarity and focus, sharpening your concentration and allowing you to fully engage in your Pilates practice with presence and intention.
- **Promote Emotional Healing:** Conscious breathing facilitates the release of emotional tension and trauma stored in the body, promoting emotional healing and fostering a greater sense of inner peace and wholeness.
- **Cultivate Mindfulness and Presence:** Conscious breathing anchors you in the present moment, enabling you to fully experience life's joys and challenges with openness, acceptance, and equanimity.

7 Breathing Exercises to Elevate Your Practice

Now that we've explored the profound advantages of conscious breathing, let's introduce seven empowering breathing exercises to integrate into your Wall Pilates practice. Each of these exercises is designed to enhance your mind-body connection, optimize your performance, and promote overall well-being. Feel free to explore these exercises at your own pace, adapting them to suit your individual needs and preferences. And remember, the key to reaping the full advantages of these exercises lies in practicing with intention, mindfulness, and compassion.

Deep Belly Breathing (Diaphragmatic Breathing):

- Lie down on your back in a comfortable position with your knees bent and your feet planted firmly on the ground.
- To begin, position one hand on your stomach and the other hand on your chest.
- Take a deep breath in through your nose, and as you are doing so, allow your stomach to expand as you fill your lungs with air.
- As you make a slow and complete exhalation via your mouth, you should feel your belly gradually falling.
- Repeat for numerous breaths, focusing on the sensation of expansion and release in your belly with each breath.

Equal Ratio Breathing (Sama Vritti):

- Sit or stand comfortably with your spine tall and shoulders relaxed.
- Begin by inhaling slowly and steadily through your nose, counting to four.
- Hold your breath for a count of four.
- Proceed to breathe out slowly and steadily through your nose, also counting to four.
- Hold your breath once more for a count of four before repeating the cycle.
- Repeat for numerous rounds, maintaining a smooth and steady rhythm.

Ocean Breath (Ujjayi Pranayama):

- Sit or stand comfortably with your spine tall and shoulders relaxed.
- Start by taking a deep inhalation through your nose, ensuring your lungs are fully filled with air.
- Then, breathe out slowly and audibly through your nose, while gently constricting the back of your throat to produce a soft, whispering sound reminiscent of ocean waves.
- Continue for numerous rounds, focusing on the soothing sound of your breath and the sensation of expansion and release in your chest.

Alternate Nostril Breathing (Nadi Shodhana):

- Settle into a comfortable position with your back straight and your shoulders relaxed.
- Make sure that your palm is pointing upward and that your left hand is resting on your left knee.
- Your right hand should be brought up to your nose, and your thumb should be placed on your right nostril, while your ring finger should be placed on your left nostril.
- Your right nostril should be closed with your thumb, and you should take a deep breath in through your left nostril.
- Your ring finger should be used to close your left nostril, and you should breathe out completely via your right nose.
- Start by taking a deep breath through your right nostril.
- The first step is to use your thumb to close your right nostril, and then breathe out completely through your left nostril.
- Keep up a smooth and consistent beat while continuing to alternate nostrils for a number of rounds.

Breathing (Relaxing Breath):

- Sit or lie comfortably with your spine tall and shoulders relaxed.
- Breathe in deeply through your nose for a count of four.
- Hold your breath for a count of seven.
- Exhale slowly and fully through your mouth for a count of eight, making a whooshing sound as you release the breath.
- Repeat for numerous rounds, allowing each exhalation to be longer and more relaxed than the last.

Box Breathing (Square Breathing):

- Sit or stand comfortably with your spine tall and shoulders relaxed.
- Take a deep inhalation through your nose, counting to four as you fill your lungs.
- Hold your breath for a count of four.
- Exhale slowly and steadily through your nose, counting to four as you release the air.
- Hold your breath for a count of four before repeating the cycle.
- Repeat for numerous rounds, visualizing the shape of a square with each inhale, hold, breathe out, and hold.

Belly Button Breathing (Hara Breathing):

- Sit or lie comfortably with your spine tall and shoulders relaxed.
- Put your hands on your belly, one hand on top of the other, with your fingertips touching your belly button.
- Breathe in deeply through your nose, letting your belly to expand and rise into your hands.
- Exhale slowly and fully through your mouth, feeling your belly gently fall away from your hands.
- Repeat for numerous rounds, focusing on the sensation of movement and rhythm in your lower abdomen.

Integrating Breathing Exercises into Your Wall Pilates Practice

Now that you've familiarized yourself with these seven empowering breathing exercises, it's time to integrate them into your Wall Pilates practice. Begin each session with a few minutes of mindful breathing to center yourself, quiet your mind, and connect with your body. Throughout your practice, continue to focus on your breath, using it as a guide to deepen your movements, enhance your awareness, and cultivate a sense of presence and intention. By integrating breathing exercises into your Wall Pilates practice, you can unlock the full potential of your body and mind, and experience profound transformation both on and off the mat.

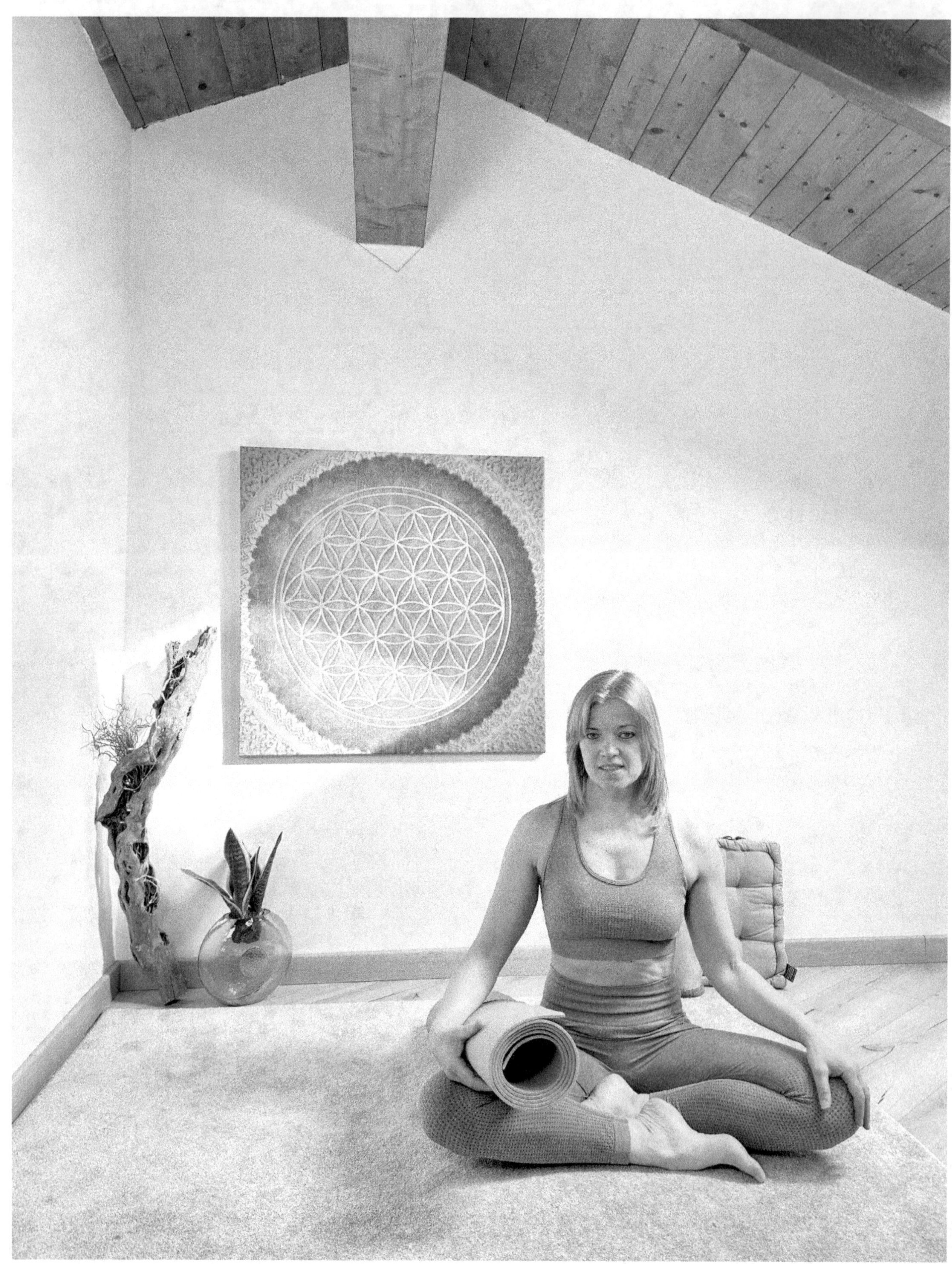

Conclusion

Congratulations on reaching the conclusion of "Wall Pilates: Transform Your Body and Mind"! You've embarked on a journey of self-discovery, strength-building, and transformation, and I'm thrilled to have been your guide along the way.

As you close the final pages of this book, I want to express my deepest gratitude for joining me on this empowering adventure. Whether you're a seasoned Pilates enthusiast or a curious beginner, I hope you've found inspiration, motivation, and practical guidance to elevate your Wall Pilates practice to new heights.

But our journey doesn't end here—it's only the beginning of a new chapter in your wellness journey. As you continue to explore and refine your Wall Pilates practice, I encourage you to embrace curiosity, self-compassion, and a spirit of adventure. Listen to your body's wisdom, honor your unique journey, and trust in your innate strength and resilience to carry you forward.

I invite you to leave feedback on Amazon and share your thoughts, insights, and experiences with fellow readers. Your feedback is invaluable and helps us continue to improve and evolve, ensuring that future readers can embark on their own transformative journeys with confidence and clarity.

As you navigate the ups and downs of life, remember that you hold the power to create the life you desire—one breath, one movement, one choice at a time. May your journey be filled with joy, vitality, and abundance, and may you continue to shine bright as you embrace the transformative power of Wall Pilates.

Wishing you a life filled with strength, vitality, and endless possibilities.

With love and gratitude,

Julia Sunnyflow

Index